THE THYROID DIET PLAN

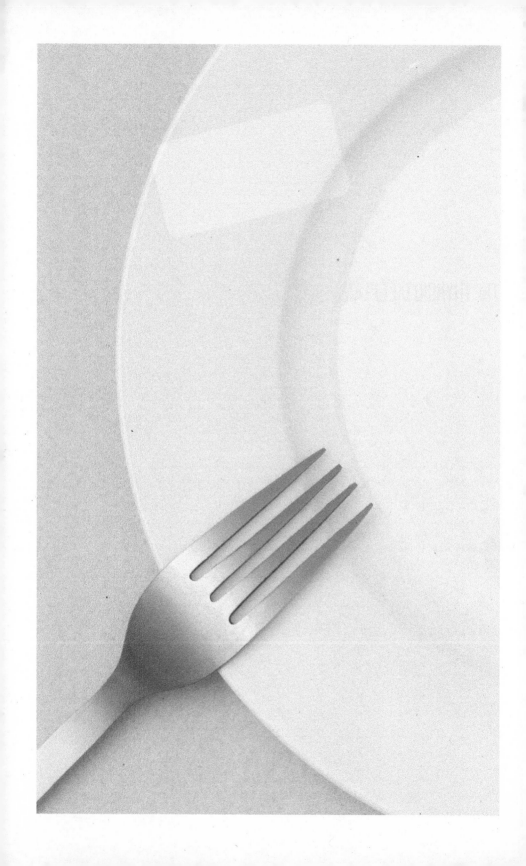

THE THYROID DIET PLAN

How to **Lose Weight, Increase Energy, and Manage Thyroid Symptoms**

HEALDSBURG
PRESS

For general information on our other products and services or to obtain technical support, please contact our Customer Care Department within the U.S. at (866) 744-2665, or outside the U.S. at (510) 253-0500.

Healdsburg Press publishes its books in a variety of electronic and print formats. Some content that appears in print may not be available in electronic books, and vice versa.

ISBN: Print 978-1-62315-236-9

Contents

Introduction

I f you are one of the 59 million Americans who suffer from some form of thyroid disease, or have a family history of thyroid problems, you may be at risk for obesity, heart disease, anxiety, depression, hair loss, and sexual dysfunction. Fortunately, the good news is that a smart diet, in combination with exercise and hormonal treatment, can help you manage these symptoms. (Be sure to consult with your physician about a course of treatment appropriate for your condition.)

This book will help you understand what's going on in your body and how to recognize the common symptoms, as well as how to improve your overall well-being with sensible exercise and delicious, healthful eating. Included here are more than 100 recipes and a 30-day meal plan to get you started on the road to better health.

Once you have the information you need to start eating right, you can take charge of your diet—and soon you'll be on your way to feeling more energetic, less anxious, and less depressed. It's the smart, healthy thing to do!

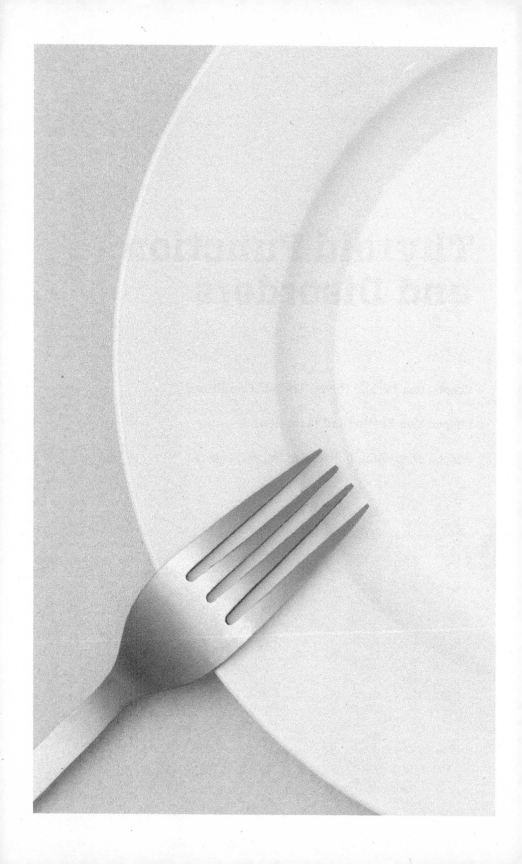

CHAPTER ONE

Do You Have a Thyroid Condition?

Symptoms of a Disorder

Signs of a thyroid condition vary from person to person and can sometimes mimic other diseases, which is one reason why thyroid disorders often remain undiagnosed. If you are experiencing symptoms that are affecting your quality of life, your physician can run some simple tests to determine whether you have a thyroid disorder. (Information about testing and what to expect can be found in chapter 2.) This chapter will focus on the function of your thyroid and the symptoms associated with the two most common disorders, hypothyroidism and hyperthyroidism.

3

Root of the Problem: Thyroid Gland

The thyroid is a large endocrine gland found in the neck, behind the thyroid cartilage, or Adam's apple. The thyroid gland has several functions, which include regulating energy use (metabolism), making proteins, and controlling the body's reaction to other hormones.

The thyroid produces hormones that regulate the rate of metabolism and affect many other systems in your body. Hormones are among the body's messengers, signaling to the cells to perform various functions. Sending messages via hormones is one way that the body maintains homeostasis, or balance.

The thyroid gland's release of hormones is regulated by thyroid-stimulating hormone (TSH), which in turn is regulated by thyrotropin-releasing hormone (TRH), a hormone produced in the hypothalamus. Many things can go wrong and disrupt this so-called feedback loop, and these events often result in hypothyroidism or hyperthyroidism. ("Hypo-" is a prefix meaning "less than normal," and "hyper-" means "greater than normal," so hypothyroidism refers to a case of a weak thyroid, whereas hyperthyroidism is a condition in which the thyroid gland becomes overactive.)

Hypothyroidism

Hypothyroidism is characterized by low levels of circulating thyroid hormones and can take several forms. Primary hypothyroidism is caused by disease of the thyroid itself. The most common cause of hypothyroidism is Hashimoto's disease, in which the body's autoimmune system attacks the thyroid gland. Women are at greater risk of developing Hashimoto's disease than men, particularly as they age. Primary hypothyroidism is also sometimes associated with other endocrine (hormonal) disorders, such as Addison's disease.

Secondary hypothyroidism refers to a problem with the feedback loop that regulates the release of thyroid hormones. Usually the problem is a deficiency of TSH, and it results from a disease of the pituitary gland or hypothalamus.

"Iatrogenic" hypothyroidism may result from removal of the thyroid gland or treatment with radioactive iodine. And if you are pregnant, you may be at risk for postpartum hypothyroidism, which is temporary.

If you answer yes to three or more of the following questions, you may be experiencing symptoms of hypothyroidism:

1. Have you been feeling unusually lethargic or fatigued despite getting enough sleep?

2. Do you find you have intolerance for cold? Are you always the chilly person in the room, unable to warm up?

3. Are you suffering from mild to moderate depression? Sadness? Are you having trouble enjoying the things you normally enjoy?

4. Is your skin unusually dry?

5. Are you battling extra pounds despite a normal diet?

6. Are you too tired to exercise?

7. Are you noticing hair loss or dry, brittle hair?

8. Does your face appear puffy?

9. Is your voice hoarse?

10. Do you have unusual muscle aches, tenderness, or stiffness?

11. Have you developed new pains, stiffness, or swelling in your joints?

12. Is your memory impaired?

13. If you are a woman, are your menstrual cycles heavier than normal, or are they irregular?

14. Have you been told you have elevated blood cholesterol?

15. Has your heart rate slowed recently, though you are not a trained athlete?

16. Do you have carpal tunnel syndrome?

Note that these symptoms may be subtle. You may have gradually become aware of feeling below par. Trust your intuition—if you're feeling that something in your body is off, it's time to seek help. If you do have hypothyroidism, your physician can help you get back on track—and rule out other serious diseases.

Low energy levels are often a symptom of poorly functioning thyroid metabolism. If you sleep eight to ten hours each night and still wake up exhausted and sluggish, you may be suffering from hypothyroidism. Another extremely troublesome yet common symptom is depression. In fact, most physicians who see patients for depression will check thyroid hormone levels first.

Some hypothyroid sufferers may notice unexpected weight gain, which only adds to their misery. If you've tried exercise and weight-loss diets and those extra pounds still won't come off, hypothyroidism could be the culprit. Other people experience hair loss on all parts of their body, including eyebrows.

You may have thought that your symptoms are a sign of aging. Although it is true that aging does affect metabolism, any unusual signs or symptoms should not be written off as "normal old age."

Hyperthyroidism

Hyperthyroidism results from the overproduction of thyroid hormones by the thyroid gland. It is usually caused by an autoimmune disorder known as Graves' disease, but occasionally it can be caused by iodine excess induced by certain drugs such as amiodarone, or by an IV contrast received in preparation for a radiographic imaging test. More unusual causes include thyroid adenomas (benign tumors) and subacute thyroiditis (inflammation of the thyroid). Sometimes, usually after giving birth, patients may have silent (or painless) thyroiditis. This temporary condition is referred to as transient hyperthyroidism, and it may transform to hypothyroidism before resolving itself.

If you answer yes to three or more of the following questions, you may have hyperthyroidism:

1. Are you always too warm, even when others in the room are comfortable?

2. Do you feel anxious or notice heart palpitations? Does your heart feel as though it's racing?

3. Are your eyeballs bulging or becoming more prominent in relation to the rest of your face?

4. Are your upper arms or thighs becoming gradually weaker?

5. Have you found yourself staring, or noticed that your eyelids take a bit too long to close?

6. If you are an older adult with coronary artery disease, have you noticed shortness of breath or chest pain increasing with exertion?

7. Do you have shortness of breath when you are lying flat in bed, or swelling in your feet and legs when you are standing or sitting?

8. Have you recently lost weight even though you haven't started a new diet or exercise program?

9. If you are a woman, have you noticed changes in your menstrual cycle?

As with hypothyroidism, these symptoms of hyperthyroidism may occur very gradually. If you are not feeling like yourself, call your doctor for further evaluation. Thyroid disease is treatable. You *can* feel better.

CHAPTER TWO

Testing and Treatment

Testing for Thyroid Disease

First, your doctor will do a physical exam, looking for signs such as lumpiness in the gland, hair loss, brittle nails, and dry skin, then will check your heart rate and probably perform an electrocardiogram (ECG).

Additionally, your doctor will draw some blood for laboratory testing. The most useful test will evaluate your levels of TSH, the hormone that stimulates thyroid function. High levels of TSH are evidence of hyperthyroidism; low levels signal hypothyroidism. Your doctor may also measure your levels of thyroid hormones, such as T3 (triiodothyronine) and T4 (thyroxine), which will help determine what type of thyroid disease you have.

Imaging studies of the thyroid gland may be ordered, and ultrasound is often used to visualize abnormalities of the thyroid, such as a goiter (lump).

Treatment for Hyperthyroidism

Some forms of hyperthyroid disease are transient (or temporary), so treatment is focused on alleviating the symptoms, typically with beta blockers (a group of drugs that work by blocking the effects of the hormone epinephrine, also known as adrenaline). Other treatments include radioactive iodine therapy and surgical subtotal thyroidectomy, which is the removal of most of the thyroid gland.

Treatment for Hypothyroidism

Hypothyroidism is easily treated with synthetic thyroid hormone supplements. The most commonly used thyroid hormone supplement is synthetic thyroxine, or

T4, in the form of tablets. Its generic name is levothyroxine, or L-thyroxine; trade names for this drug in the United States include Synthroid, Levothroid, and Levoxyl. Tirosint is a relatively new formulation of levothyroxine in a liquid gelcap.

Most doctors recommend brand-name supplemental T4 instead of generic because there have been reports of broad variations in the actual amount of T4 in some generic tablets.

A less commonly used medication is synthetic triiodothyronine, or T3, known generically as liothyronine and sold under the brand name Cytomel. In recent years physicians have begun to prescribe T3 in addition to T4.

A synthetic T4/T3 combination tablet manufactured under the brand name Thyrolar (generic name liotrix) has been developed, but it is not often used in the United States, at least in part due to its short supply.

Before synthetic forms of thyroid hormone became available in the 1950s, dessicated porcine thyroid hormone was used to treat patients with hypothyroid disease. This medication is prepared from pig thyroid glands and is enjoying a resurgence today among holistically oriented physicians who believe that it resolves symptoms better than synthetic hormones. Available by prescription, brand names include Nature-Throid, Westhroid-P, and Armour Thyroid.

The latest guidelines for the treatment of thyroid disease, published in 2012, remain controversial among physicians and their patients. These guidelines recommend relying solely on the test for TSH to diagnose hypothyroid disease. However, many physicians today believe that other factors should be considered, including the amount of circulating T3 and T4 and any thyroid autoantibodies present in the blood.

. Another controversial guideline is the recommendation that patients with hypothyroidism be treated with T4 supplements only. This guideline ignores the results of several large studies, especially a 2009 Danish study, which showed that 49 percent of patients felt better with a combination therapy of T3 and T4.

The guidelines go on to say that dessicated porcine thyroid hormone should not be used for the treatment of hypothyroidism, as there is no evidence to support its efficacy when compared with levothyroxine. There is, however, plenty of anecdotal evidence that it works. You should ask your doctor what studies he or she is basing your treatment on before you start a regimen of thyroid replacement, and have a frank conversation about other treatment options.

Taking Your Medication

There are a few things you should know about taking your medication properly. Taking thyroid hormone on an empty stomach and waiting at least one hour before eating has a significant effect on absorption. It is critical to stick to this rule in order to realize the full benefit of your dosage. Also, if you make a drastic change to the amount of fiber in your diet, get your thyroid hormone levels checked again, as fiber affects absorption.

Avoid taking other medications or supplements within three hours of taking your thyroid replacement hormone. Some antidepressants can change the effectiveness of thyroid hormones, so be very careful when taking drugs such as Prozac or Zoloft. Be sure your doctor is aware of all the medications and supplements you are currently taking.

Thyroid hormone replacement is a lifelong commitment, and you can't stop while pregnant or breastfeeding. If you have concerns, discuss them with your ob-gyn, but don't just stop taking your pills.

Your thyroid function may change over time, and the dosage of your medication may need to be adjusted accordingly. Once you start treatment, you should see your doctor once a year to check your hormone levels—and at any time if you begin to feel sluggish, depressed, or bloated. If your doctor does not take your concerns seriously, or fails to address them adequately, seek a second opinion. This is a quality-of-life issue and should not be treated lightly.

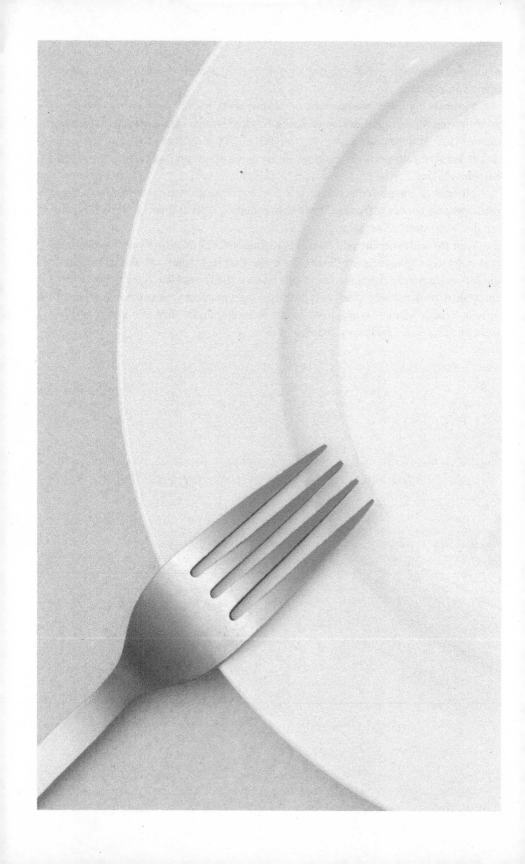

CHAPTER THREE

Metabolism and Related Issues

What Is Metabolism?

Metabolism is a series of chemical reactions that take place in the cells of every living organism to produce energy. Humans and other animals metabolize three major groups of nutrients—carbohydrates, fats (also known as lipids), and proteins—which we derive from food. We also need a number of vitamins and minerals to help us with the metabolic process. In order to have a healthy metabolism, your diet should reflect your body's special needs.

Genetics versus the Environment

When you think of metabolism, you may think of how quickly you gain or lose weight. Metabolism directly influences the rate at which we burn calories, so the issue of metabolic rate is what most of us focus on as we try to gain or lose weight, or as we wonder about our energy levels when compared to other people's. This part of metabolism is genetically programmed, but it is also influenced by environment. That is, you can boost your metabolism through changes in diet, exercise, and other lifestyle habits.

Toxins

Every day we are exposed to toxins in pesticides, food additives, tobacco, alcohol, industrial chemicals, and even toxic substances formed through the metabolism of our diets, which may be inefficiently eliminated by our bodies. These toxins are stored in the fat cells of the body.

Some studies have found a link between environmental toxins and thyroid hormones. Other studies suggest that the rate at which the body excretes residual environmental toxins during weight loss can have a detrimental effect on your metabolism: As you lose weight, your fat cells shrink, and the toxins that are stored there are released into your bloodstream. If you have a high body mass index (BMI), you have a high proportion of fat to muscle. Since toxins are stored in the fat cells, that means you have a large repository of toxins in your body. (To calculate your BMI and find out what your score means, use the easy calculator provided online by the National Institutes of Health.)

Toxins affect our ability to produce energy from fat. Not only do toxins reduce the level of thyroid hormones—which, as we have discussed, regulate the level of metabolism—but they also weaken a special coenzyme that is needed to lose weight.

Detoxification is an important concept in health maintenance, and we'll discuss it further in chapter 4.

Stress

In a stressful or threatening situation, your body instinctively reacts with a fight-or-flight response, a "high alert" condition during which you feel the rush of adrenaline. In the wild, this response would help you attack your prey or escape from danger, but in the modern world this response may be triggered on a daily basis by all kinds of stresses. Fight-or-flight is triggered any time your sympathetic nervous system is stimulated, resulting in the release of a hormone called cortisol. Although this response is useful in the short term, its long-term consequences are severe, because cortisol suppresses your immune system and slows your digestive processes. An excess of cortisol can cause weight gain, hypertension, diabetes, and depression.

Cardiovascular exercise and meditation can reduce stress and its negative effects on your body, so they're well worth the effort.

Insomnia

Millions of Americans suffer from insomnia, which has a variety of negative consequences related to metabolism. Studies have shown that insomnia is related to thyroid function and has a negative effect on the feedback loop among the hypothalamus, pituitary, and adrenal glands.

Insomnia affects cortisol concentrations and impaired glucose tolerance as well. All these factors contribute to weight gain. The good news is that by adhering to good sleep habits—for example, going to bed in a darkened room at approximately the same time each night—you can improve your sleep in many natural ways.

Lack of sleep has many harmful effects on your metabolism. If your insomnia is persistent, you should discuss this condition with your physician.

Nutritional Deficiencies

Since a healthy metabolism relies on breaking down nutrients in order to produce energy, good nutrition is key. If you fail to take in an adequate amount of key nutrients, your metabolism won't function in a healthy manner.

In addition to energy, your body needs different substances to build and repair its tissues and to produce various proteins, hormones, and enzymes. You also need plenty of water to keep everything running smoothly, so be sure you are always well hydrated.

When you begin to watch your nutrient intake, you should have a clear understanding of the foods you take in. Let's start with carbohydrates. There are three different forms of carbohydrates: starch, sugar, and fiber. Starch and sugar are a major source of energy for humans, and fiber provides bulk, which is healthy for your colon. Foods that are primarily carbohydrates include potatoes, pasta, bread, and rice.

We also need protein in our diets. Proteins are made up of amino acids. Amino acids are sometimes called the "building blocks of life" and are needed to carry out energy production and almost every other bodily or cellular function. Protein is found in eggs, meat, fish, dairy products, soy, and legumes.

Fats produce twice as much energy as carbohydrates or protein. Fats are important nutrients, as they help form cellular structure, absorb fat-soluble vitamins, and provide reserve energy storage. Essential fatty acids for your metabolism can be found in fish, walnuts and almonds, and dark leafy greens.

Although minerals and vitamins don't directly produce energy, they are necessary components of the metabolic pathways of the body. Specific minerals and vitamins that are essential to a healthy metabolism are discussed in chapter 5.

Food Allergies

If you have trouble with your weight, you may have a food allergy or intolerance that is contributing to a sluggish metabolism. Food allergies can cause water retention and weight gain because you may be unable to completely digest the food, and because allergens cause inflammation, which your body will try to reduce by diluting the offending material in water.

Partially digested foods in your colon can also result in cravings and food addictions. You may get a "high" from eating the food allergen, but when it wears off, you will crave it again. This can lead to binge eating of the very foods to which you have an intolerance, creating a vicious cycle that includes weight gain and decreased metabolism.

Determining what foods you're allergic to may help you overcome cravings and get rid of bloating and water retention. Additionally, avoiding your food allergens can boost your metabolism and your body's ability to burn fat. Many people who have investigated their food allergies have improved their quality of life tremendously by identifying and eliminating these foods from their diets.

PART TWO

The Thyroid Weight-Loss Plan

Chapter Four Sensible Weight Loss

Chapter Five The Food Checklist

Chapter Six The 30-Day Meal Plan

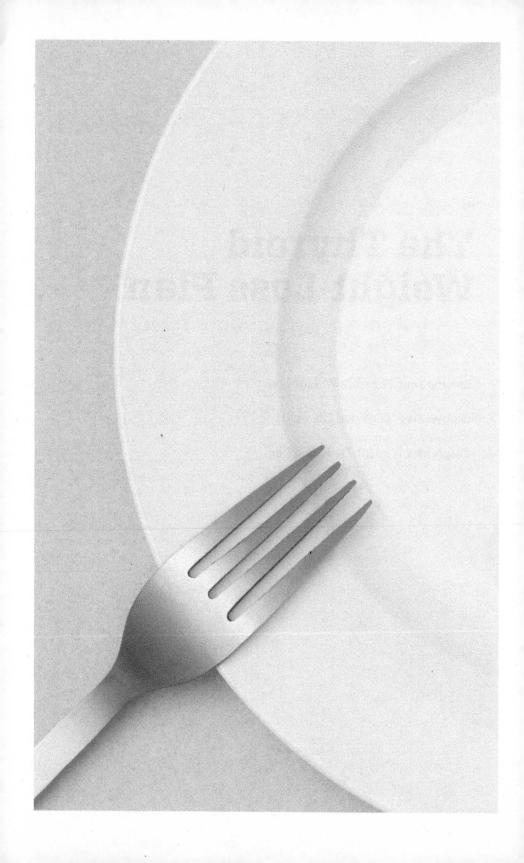

Sensible Weight Loss

Metabolism and Hunger

Perhaps you've recently experienced a weight gain, and you're wondering why. Or you have been struggling with your weight for years, but your metabolism just keeps slowing down. Some physicians believe that when people have a chronic weight problem, their bodies continue to establish new "set points" for weight; as their weight increases, their metabolism slows. They may consume fewer calories in an attempt to lose weight, but their body burns those calories at a slower rate in order to maintain their weight.

17

Unfortunately, a decreased metabolism does not necessarily affect your sense of hunger. Normally, when you consume an adequate amount of carbs, your hypothalamus releases a neurotransmitter called serotonin, which results in a feeling of fullness. If you have thyroid disease, your metabolism is slowed down, but your brain still perceives a need for food intake. This need is greater than your metabolism can process successfully, which results in weight gain.

As you keep gaining weight due to your hypothyroidism-affected metabolism, you may experience insulin resistance. Insulin is a hormone produced in the pancreas that controls the absorption of blood glucose (sugar) into the cells. When you eat carbs, your body digests them into simple sugars, which enter the bloodstream. As the level of simple sugars in your blood increases, the pancreas releases insulin to help clear the sugar out of the bloodstream and into your cells.

When the cells become overwhelmed with too much sugar over the course of years or even decades, eventually they lose sensitivity to insulin and cannot continue to absorb the blood sugar, leaving higher and higher concentrations of sugar in the bloodstream. Ironically, because your cells are not getting the blood sugar they need, your pancreas will release more insulin (hyperinsulinemia) and your body will crave more carbs, which in turn increases your blood sugar levels (hyperglycemia), in a vicious circle that, if left untreated, will result in type 2 diabetes.

Insulin resistance also prevents your body from utilizing stored fat for energy, another cause of weight gain, or resistance to weight loss. Insulin resistance–based hyperglycemia and hyperinsulinemia are associated with an increased risk of high cholesterol, coronary artery disease, and high blood pressure.

At the opposite extreme, the resulting high levels of insulin can result in low blood sugar—yet another potential hazard for people with hypothyroidism.

The good news is that you can plan a healthy diet that is very satisfying, with an emphasis on chicken, fish, fruits and vegetables without starch, legumes, and whole grains. Your cravings for carbs will be dramatically reduced with a diet plan focused on foods with a low glycemic index—foods that do not dramatically raise the amount of glucose in your blood—and your insulin resistance will be reduced or eliminated.

There are specific foods that will help your thyroid function more efficiently. The meal plan and recipes in the next few chapters will guide you to the most efficient way to naturally reduce insulin resistance and increase the effectiveness of your thyroid gland or your thyroid hormone replacement supplements.

A New Approach to Dieting

There is only one way to lose weight: Burn more energy than you take in through calories. If your body doesn't utilize the calories you take in through your diet, they are stored as fat.

Unfortunately, if you have hypothyroid disease, your body will utilize fewer of the calories you take in through your diet, and the rest will be stored as fat. Knowing this, you may feel that you are at a disadvantage when it comes to losing weight. However, if you have seen your doctor and are on a thyroid supplement, your body is normalizing, and you will be able to jump-start your metabolism through a balanced low-calorie diet and exercise program.

The average person expends 2,000 calories per day, and there are 3,500 calories in a pound of fat. Thus, in order to lose a pound of fat in one week, you would have to expend 500 more calories than you take in each day. That would mean you should target your diet plan to 1,500 calories per day.

But not everyone expends 2,000, calories per day. Your total daily calorie expenditure equals the calories used for your normal bodily functions (breathing, sleeping, keeping your heart beating), your exercise calories, and your digestion calories. This represents the number of calories needed to maintain your weight. One way to calculate how many calories you should have in your diet each day is to know your basal metabolic rate (BMR).

A quick way to estimate your BMR is to take your body weight in pounds and multiply it by 10. Say you weigh 140 pounds; then your BMR would be 1,400 calories. The second factor to consider is the number of calories you use in physical activity each day. Consider the following four levels of activity:

Sedentary (sitting most of the day): 20%

Lightly active (daily chores, some walking): 37.5%

Moderately active (constantly moving, exercising daily): 40%

Very active (heavy exercise for long periods of training): 50%

Multiply your BMR by the appropriate percentage, and add that number to your BMR. So, if you are moderately active, you would calculate that 40 percent of 1,400 is 560, and 1,400 + 560 = 1,960. Finally, factor in the calories you use during digestion, which are estimated at 10 percent of your BMR + activity level. In our example, 10 percent of 1,960 is 196, so you would need to take in 1,960 + 196 = 2,156 calories per day in order to maintain your weight.

In addition to weight, BMR is also linked to your age, height, and gender; there are BMR calculators available online that will also take into account these factors and help you determine a more accurate BMR. This calculation will result in a daily calorie budget that will enable you to maintain, gain, or lose weight. As always, for each pound you want to lose, you have to take in 3,500 less calories than you expend.

Exercise

Exercise burns calories efficiently, and it revs up your metabolism. An effective exercise plan includes both cardiovascular exercise and strength training.

The benefits of cardiovascular exercise are many: lower blood sugar levels, decreased circulating insulin, decreased insulin resistance, boosted metabolism, decreased cholesterol, and lower rates of cardiovascular disease and diabetes.

Strength training is also an exceptionally important part of any exercise routine. Muscle cells have a higher metabolic rate than fat cells, so your metabolism will increase as you gain muscle mass.

Exercise does not require any special equipment or gym membership. You can begin with a brisk 15-minute walk after supper, at least three times per week. It is essential to elevate your heart rate to get the cardiovascular benefit, so do walk quickly—you should be able to walk a mile in 15 minutes, and you should aim for a shorter time as you become more fit. It can be fun to walk with a friend, and having an exercise partner is a good motivator. Eventually, you will be able to increase the amount of aerobic exercise you do each week. Low-intensity, prolonged exercise (45 minutes or more) has been associated with reduced insulin resistance.

Bicycling is also good aerobic exercise, as is dancing—when you're home alone, turn up the volume on your stereo, or on your computer speakers by connecting to an online music services (YouTube, Pandora, Spotify, and the iTunes store, to name a few). Aim for at least 15 minutes of solid aerobic exercise at a time.

If you have the time and money, joining a gym is a great way to jump-start your exercise routine, especially if you join with a friend. Most gyms offer a variety of aerobic classes, or classes that combine aerobic exercise with strength training, such as Pilates, Zumba, kickboxing, cycling, or belly dancing.

Strength training can be very simple, as you can use the weight of your own body to build up selected muscle groups. Some examples of exercises to try on your own include push-ups, pull-ups, squats, and lunges. You can purchase handheld weights from 5 to 8 pounds each to do some simple curls to tone your arms and build more muscle.

Avoiding Toxins

As we discussed in chapter 3, toxins affect your metabolism in an unhealthy way. As you begin your diet plan, consider detoxification, which is an essential component of maintaining health.

We are exposed constantly to toxins, in the pesticides in our foods, in the chemicals we use to clean our homes, and in the pollutants in our air and water. A stunning example of just how toxic we have become was revealed in a study at the Stanford University Hospital, which found that newborn babies had high levels of many toxins in their first stool. The mothers' bodies were overloaded with toxic substances, which crossed the placental barrier and caused newborns to have toxic levels of mercury, lead, and even DDT (a pesticide outlawed decades ago) in their first stool.

A study at Mt. Sinai School of Medicine, performed by collecting blood and urine in a small sample of patients, found 167 different chemicals in the body fluids, including an average of 91 industrial chemicals in each person.

The National Institutes of Health and the National Cancer Institute, in a study of cancer and the environment, hypothesized that two-thirds of all cancers could be linked to environmental toxins. Toxins are also linked to autoimmune diseases, many of which affect the thyroid gland. Mercury and lead, trace metals that serve no nutritional purpose, can build up if your body's detoxification system is not functioning properly and can cause many harmful and chronic health conditions.

To begin to understand how toxins affect the body, let's first discuss how your body accumulates toxins. External toxins are taken in through air, water, and food. Internal toxins are the by-products of the food we've digested and metabolized. The body has a system in place to process and expel ingested or inhaled toxins, but it may malfunction and result in toxin buildup over a period of time. Eventually these toxins will permeate the cellular barrier of the gut, affecting the body's cellular metabolism and impacting critical organ systems.

As we saw in chapter 3, carbohydrates turn to glucose, proteins to amino acids, and fats to fatty acids. Each of these conversion processes results in natural toxins, which, in the normal course of events, should be eliminated by the natural digestive process.

But when the food we eat is composed largely of nonnutritional and processed substances, the digestive system, particularly the liver, gets overwhelmed and is no longer able to process and eliminate these harmful substances. If our toxic load becomes too great, toxins will be absorbed through the gut and stored in various cell types.

There are many reasons for such a failure, but most are consequences of our modern lifestyle. Stress affects the autonomic nervous system, which controls bowel mobility. High levels of stress upset the natural interaction of the parasympathetic and sympathetic nervous systems, which control blood supply of the bowel. Inadequate chewing and consumption of processed foods contribute to inadequate digestion.

Constipation is both a symptom and a cause of toxic bowel health. Digested food should be liquid when it enters the large intestine. If it is not, it will block further action in the small and large intestines until it is eliminated. Retained waste—mostly bacteria—will remain in the bowel and prevent adequate digestion of subsequent meals, causing gas, bloating, weight gain, inflammation, skin disorders, headaches, and joint and muscle pain.

The body can become inflamed, due to the imbalance of the microorganisms that allow the gut to function properly, which can eventually affect the entire immune system. This is a frequent cause of autoimmune illness, including many severe rheumatologic diseases and various types of thyroid disease.

Parasites may also cause toxicity. It is estimated that one-third of the American population is infected with intestinal parasites, particularly *Giardia*. Intestinal parasites can cause constipation, diarrhea, bloating, and abnormal stools. *Candida* (yeast) and parasitic infections may contribute to leaky gut, a condition in which the porous lining of the intestine absorbs toxins from the gut into the bloodstream.

The liver is of critical importance in detoxification. Anything absorbed from the intestine must pass through the bloodstream to the liver. The liver depends on proper nutrients and amino acids to perform its specific digestive functions and its control of blood glucose. For example, the liver produces bile, which is needed for the elimination of toxins. If the liver is overwhelmed, it becomes slow in all functions, including bile production. Even with adequate production of bile, if you don't take in enough fiber to absorb the toxins in the bowel and eliminate them through normal bowel movements, they will be reabsorbed into the gut and deposited in tissues throughout the body by the bloodstream.

Vitamins and Supplements

Many supplements interfere with the absorption of thyroid supplements, so if you are taking supplemental thyroid hormone, consider possible interactions. Both calcium and chromium picolinate supplements, for example, have been shown to interfere with absorption of thyroid medications, so it's wise to take these supplements at least four hours before or after your thyroid medicine.

Coffee also lowers absorption of thyroid medication, as do fiber supplements—these should be taken at least two hours before or after your thyroid medication.

Although natural flavonoids, found in vegetables, fruits, and tea, are thought to have possible cardiovascular benefits, flavonoid supplements in high doses may suppress the function of the thyroid gland and should thus be avoided.

CHAPTER FIVE

The Food Checklist

Beneficial Foods

Throughout history, people have learned through trial and error the health benefits of various nutritional supplements and foods. Chinese medicine, for example, is based on the therapeutic use of traditional herbs and foods. Our society is once again learning to become attuned to the special properties of many foods as they relate to disease and health.

Thyroid disease has existed as long as people have had thyroid glands; before thyroid hormone supplements were available, people learned what types of foods helped them to function better. There is strong evidence that these foods can help you with your thyroid problem.

With the weight gain associated with hypothyroid disease, the single biggest factor in planning your thyroid diet should be calorie control, followed by control of your carbs. You should be eating a minimal amount of processed foods, which are full of toxins. Center your diet on nonstarchy vegetables, lean meats, legumes, fiber for colon health, and increased fluid intake. Fruits, nuts, heart-healthy fats, and omega-3 fatty acids should all be emphasized, as they prevent illnesses associated with thyroid disease (such as heart disease, diabetes, cancer, and other autoimmune diseases). Eliminating toxins will lower the body's level of inflammation, which is a key factor in some of these illnesses.

Vitamins and Minerals to Include in Your Diet

The following vitamins and minerals have been shown to improve thyroid health. However, be aware that dosage is important. Taking too high a dose can result in unwelcome side effects. When in doubt, be sure to consult with your physician.

Iodine is a vital nutrient that is essential to thyroid function. Although most thyroid disease in the United States is due to autoimmune disorders, the greatest cause of thyroid disease worldwide is lack of iodine. In the United States, iodine deficiency is rare because of the use of iodized salt since the 1920s. Supplemental iodine should always be taken with care, as extra iodine could cause a flare-up of Hashimoto's disease by stimulating autoimmune antibodies. Fish, dairy products, and grains are good natural sources of iodine.

Vitamin D is an essential nutrient, and deficiency of vitamin D has been linked to Hashimoto's disease, which causes hypothyroidism. One study revealed that more than 90 percent of patients with Hashimoto's were deficient in vitamin D, although causality is not clear. Hyperthyroid disease, including Graves' disease, causes bone loss, which is exacerbated by low levels of vitamin D. When hyperthyroidism is treated, bone mass is reestablished, for which vitamin D is important. Foods that are good sources of vitamin D include mushrooms, eggs, dairy products, and fatty fish. Sunlight is an important source of vitamin D. Any vitamin D supplementation should be taken in consultation with your physician.

Selenium is a trace mineral found within the thyroid gland, and it is a critical component in thyroid function. Studies have showed that selenium has a beneficial effect on the amount of thyroid antibody found in patients with Hashimoto's disease—and on their mood. Other benefits of selenium include boosting the immune system, improving cognitive function, and increasing fertility in men and women. In fact, placebo-controlled studies have shown that selenium is associated with an overall decrease in mortality rate. However, be aware that excess selenium can cause GI problems and can potentially raise the risk of type 2 diabetes and cancer, so again, it is important to undertake supplementation of your diet with the guidance of your physician. Good dietary sources of selenium include tuna, crab, lobster, and Brazil nuts.

Vitamin B$_{12}$ has beneficial effects on mood and on the nervous system; a B$_{12}$ deficiency can lead to irreversible neurologic effects, so patients with thyroid disease should routinely be tested for B$_{12}$ deficiency. Good sources of B$_{12}$ include sardines, salmon, liver, meat, dairy products, fortified cereals, and nutritional yeast.

Vitamin C has a beneficial effect on thyroid health. Good sources of vitamin C are parsley and other herbs, hot and sweet peppers, citrus fruits, and leafy greens.

Foods to Avoid

When considering your diet plan, it is also important to consider foods that can cause problems for your thyroid.

Some foods, called goitrogens, release a compound called goitrin when they are broken down by the digestive system. Goitrin may interfere with the synthesis of hormones produced by the thyroid gland, especially if coupled with an iodine deficiency. However, heating goitrogenic vegetables, which include broccoli, cabbage, and cauliflower, usually mitigates this effect. Other goitrogenic foods include peaches, horseradish, mustard, mustard greens, radishes, spinach, rutabagas, turnips, cassava root, and kale.

Another food that's potentially goitrogenic is soy. This is somewhat controversial, since people with adequate iodine stores don't become hypothyroid by consuming soy. However, certain compounds in soy can interfere with the synthesis of thyroid hormone. If you have hypothyroidism, you should eat soy only in moderation.

Millet, a grain, is a food to avoid if you are hypothyroid. It appears to suppress thyroid function in people who have adequate iodine stores.

Fluoride in tap water has also been implicated as a suppressor of thyroid hormone. You might want to consider drinking and cooking with purified or bottled water if you are suffering from thyroid disease.

Making the Right Diet Choices

You don't need to worry about taking a lot of supplements. Many of the nutrients you need to maximize your thyroid health can be found in foods readily available at your local supermarket.

First, as noted above, processed foods, though full of iodized salt, are generally not healthy. A better option is to prepare your own simple meals, flavoring your foods as needed with iodized salt.

Fish is a good source of iodine, vitamin B_{12}, and vitamin D, and the fatty fishes—such as tuna, salmon, trout, and sardines—are a good source of selenium. Some healthy prepared foods may be available at your supermarket's seafood counter, such as steamed fish, crab, or lobster. Canned sardines are a tasty snack and, like tuna, promote good thyroid function.

Whole grains are a better source of fiber than simple carbohydrates, and they are a good source of both iodine and B_{12}; they can be found in bagels, breads, crackers, and pastas.

Dairy is important in your diet if you have thyroid disorder, as dairy products are an excellent source of vitamin D. However, if you are attempting to lose any weight you have gained from thyroid disease, look for low-fat dairy products.

Nuts are a good source of many nutrients, including vitamin B_{12} and selenium. Cruciferous vegetables (such as broccoli, cabbage, and cauliflower), peaches, and pears, should be avoided, but other fruits and vegetables are excellent. Dressing made with cold-pressed olive oil added to a healthy salad is a delightful source of nutrition and will provide a boost to your metabolism.

To help you make the right diet choices, follow the 30-day meal plan provided in chapter 6, and remember to keep portion sizes reasonable. As long as you regularly take your hormone supplements and stick with your new diet and fitness plan, you can be sure to regain your energy and good health.

CHAPTER SIX

The 30-Day Meal Plan

This low-calorie, low-carbohydrate diet plan is designed to help you shed the pounds you've gained due to your thyroid disorder. The menu options provided here are meant to help you plan your meals, but you may certainly substitute preferred items according to your tastes—one fruit for another, for instance.

Remember, dieting does not mean skipping meals. Breakfast, in particular, is considered by some to be the most important meal of the day, and missing breakfast will actually slow down your metabolism, because your body will go into starvation mode and will begin to conserve calories.

Also keep in mind that you need to watch your portions. A good rule of thumb to follow is that a portion is the size that will fit in the palm of your hand. This will help you maintain a healthy caloric intake without having to count calories.

Most of the items listed in the meal plan are included in part 3 (you will notice that they are marked with a *). In addition to the breakfast, lunch, and dinner entrées, you may eat two snacks per day. During the first stage of your diet, when you're still losing weight, stick to four whole-grain Triscuits or other wheat crackers, a piece of fruit, or some raw vegetables seasoned with lemon juice. When you've reached your desired weight, you can begin incorporating the savory snacks and desserts listed in chapters 10 and 11, but remember to do so in moderation.

Day 1 *Breakfast*: Asparagus-Tomato Frittata*
Lunch: grilled chicken, Seaweed Salad*, watermelon chunks
Dinner: grilled halibut, quinoa, green beans, applesauce

Day 2 *Breakfast*: Mediterranean Scrambled Eggs with Garlic and Basil*
Lunch: tuna salad, celery sticks with peanut butter
Dinner: Apple Couscous with Curry*, asparagus, melon wedge

Day 3 *Breakfast*: granola with cottage cheese, orange slices
Lunch: Endive with Shrimp*, apple slices
Dinner: Burgundy Salmon*, green beans with dill

Day 4 *Breakfast*: Poached Egg and Toast*, applesauce
Lunch: grilled chicken, quinoa, orange slices
Dinner: Grilled Herbed Tuna*, asparagus

Day 5 *Breakfast*: Egg Muffins "On the Go"*, berries
Lunch: Crunchy Pea and Barley Salad*, chopped apples and raisins
Dinner: Baked Salmon with Capers and Olives*, green salad with red onions

Day 6 *Breakfast*: Spicy Scrambled Eggs*, bacon, melon wedge
Lunch: Southwestern Quinoa and Black Bean Salad* on lettuce bed
Dinner: grilled chicken, Rosemary-Roasted Acorn Squash*, green salad with cucumbers and red onions, chopped apples and raisins

Day 7 *Breakfast*: Blueberry-Cherry Parfait*
Lunch: Smoky Black Bean Burgers*, tomato slices
Dinner: Poached Cod*, zucchini and yellow squash, orange slices

Day 8 *Breakfast*: Mung Bean Porridge*, melon wedge
Lunch: Open-Faced Eggplant Parmesan Sandwiches*, berries
Dinner: Herb-Marinated Flounder*, green salad, apple slices with cinnamon

Day 9 *Breakfast*: Spicy Scrambled Eggs*, bacon, sliced tomatoes
Lunch: Mediterranean Tuna Salad Sandwiches*
Dinner: Roasted Sea Bass*, orange slices

Day 10 *Breakfast*: Brazil Nut and Banana Breakfast Smoothie*
Lunch: Turkish Lentil Soup*, green beans
Dinner: Chermoula Salmon*, berries

Day 11 *Breakfast*: Breakfast Tuna Melt*
Lunch: Open-Faced Grilled Caesar Salad Sandwiches*, chopped apples and raisins
Dinner: Balsamic-Glazed Salmon*, quinoa, green peas, cantaloupe wedge

Day 12 *Breakfast*: Blueberry-Avocado Smoothie*
Lunch: Moroccan Tomato and Roasted Pepper Salad with Grilled Chicken*
Dinner: grilled halibut, Italian Mushroom-Stuffed Zucchini*,
orange slices

Day 13 *Breakfast*: Egg Muffins "On the Go"*, berries
Lunch: Farro Bean Soup*, green salad
Dinner: Cod Gratin*, green beans with dill, sliced tomatoes,
melon wedge

Day 14 *Breakfast*: Super Avocado and Honey Smoothie*, berries
Lunch: grilled chicken, Cold Cucumber Soup*, melon wedge
Dinner: Sweet Roasted Beet Salad with Oranges and Onions*, feta cheese,
baked apple

Day 15 *Breakfast*: Poached Egg and Toast*, melon wedge
Lunch: Greek Roasted Red Pepper and Feta Soup*, green salad
Dinner: Grilled Eggplant Pesto Stack*, green pea and corn succotash,
apple slices

Day 16 *Breakfast*: Blueberry-Cherry Parfait*
Lunch: Garden Salad with Sardine Fillets*
Dinner: Baked Ziti*, green salad

Day 17 *Breakfast*: Fresh Veggie Frittata*
Lunch: Four-Bean Salad* on bed of greens, orange slices
Dinner: Hearty Clam Spaghetti*, green salad with avocado

Day 18 *Breakfast*: Greek Eggs and Potatoes*, banana
Lunch: grilled salmon, Asparagus Salad*
Dinner: Eggplant and Tomato Ragu*, green salad, apple slices

Day 19 *Breakfast*: Blueberry-Banana Smoothie*
Lunch: Italian Cream of Mushroom Soup with Red Wine*, sliced tomatoes
Dinner: Hearty Shrimp Salad*, lemon asparagus

Day 20 *Breakfast*: Eggs with Asparagus Soldiers*
Lunch: Zuppa di Fagioli*, tomatoes on greens
Dinner: Grilled Herbed Tuna*, green salad with olives and tomatoes,
apple slices

Day 21 *Breakfast*: Cinnamon Quinoa with Blueberries*
Lunch: Provençal Shrimp Soup with Leeks and Fennel*, tomato slices
Dinner: Grilled Eggplant Pesto Stack*, green beans, banana

Day 22 *Breakfast*: Power-Packed Banana-Quinoa Smoothie*
Lunch: Moroccan Tomato Soup*, orange slices
Dinner: Seasoned Root Vegetables*, green salad with hard-boiled eggs, apple slices

Day 23 *Breakfast*: Quick Chocolate-Banana Smoothie*
Lunch: grilled chicken, Raw Zucchini Salad*
Dinner: Poached Cod*, green peas, quinoa

Day 24 *Breakfast*: Blueberry-Banana Smoothie*
Lunch: Caprese Panini*, lemon asparagus
Dinner: Bouillabaisse*, green salad, orange slices

Day 25 *Breakfast*: Poached Egg and Toast*, melon wedge
Lunch: Korean Seaweed Soup*, green salad with tomatoes
Dinner: Stuffed Bell Peppers*, quinoa, baked apple

Day 26 *Breakfast*: Healthier Banana Bread*
Lunch: Perfect Summer Ratatouille*, green salad
Dinner: Grilled Herbed Tuna*, roasted sweet potatoes, green peas, berries

Day 27 *Breakfast*: Blueberry-Cherry Parfait*
Lunch: Turkish Lentil Soup*, yellow squash and zucchini
Dinner: Eggplant and Tomato Ragu*, braised endive, melon wedge

Day 28 *Breakfast*: Italian Eggs with Tomatoes*
Lunch: Greek Roasted Red Pepper and Feta Soup*, green salad
Dinner: Herb-Marinated Flounder*, lemon asparagus, sliced tomatoes

Day 29 *Breakfast*: Power-Packed Banana-Quinoa Smoothie*
Lunch: Open-Faced Eggplant Parmesan Sandwiches*, green salad
Dinner: Poached Cod*, asparagus, baked apple

Day 30 *Breakfast*: Egg Muffins "On the Go"*, melon wedge
Lunch: Endive with Shrimp*, apple slices
Dinner: Roasted Sea Bass*, quinoa, zucchini

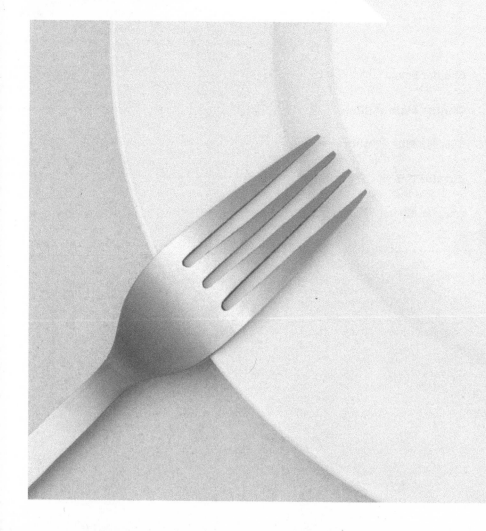

CHAPTER SEVEN

Breakfast

Smoked Salmon and Egg English Muffin

An English muffin topped with eggs and smoked salmon makes a hearty, delicious breakfast. Salmon is a great source of omega-3 fatty acids, which improve the cardiovascular system. Both tomatoes and salmon contain high amounts of selenium, which specifically benefit the thyroid.

¼ teaspoon olive oil
4 egg whites, lightly beaten
2 tomato slices
2 ounces smoked salmon
2 whole-wheat English muffins, split and toasted
Capers (optional)
Iodized table salt and freshly ground black pepper

Heat the oil in a small nonstick skillet over medium heat. Add the egg whites. Stir constantly until set, about 1 minute.

Layer the egg whites, tomato slices, and salmon on the English muffin bottoms. Add a few capers, if desired. Season with salt and pepper and cover with the muffin tops. Serve warm.

Breakfast Tuna Melt

SERVES 2

Although tuna melts may not come to mind when you're thinking of breakfast, this light version is a nice start to the day. Tuna, like many fish, offers iodine, which is helpful to those with hypothyroidism. Substituting avocado for the usual mayonnaise not only provides healthier fats but also creates a more complex taste.

One 5-ounce can tuna packed in water, drained
¼ cup diced celery
1 tablespoon minced red onion
2 whole-wheat English muffins, split
1 tablespoon mashed avocado
2 tomato slices
2 low-fat cheese slices
Iodized table salt and freshly ground black pepper

Combine the tuna, celery, and onion in a medium bowl.

Coat a large skillet with cooking spray and place it over low heat. Place the English muffins in the pan. Spread the mashed avocado on the two muffin bottoms, then top each with a slice of tomato, half of the tuna mixture, and a slice of cheese. Season with salt and pepper.

Cook until the cheese melts and the English muffins are toasted, about 2 minutes. Place the English muffin tops over the sandwiches. Serve immediately.

Asparagus-Tomato Frittata

Asparagus and tomatoes are both excellent sources of selenium, which helps regulate thyroid function and improves the immune system. This dish is both a hearty and healthy way to start the day.

2 eggs
4 tablespoons plain nonfat yogurt
Pinch of iodized table salt
1 tablespoon butter
½ cup sliced asparagus (1-inch pieces)
1 medium plum tomato, diced

Preheat the broiler.

Beat the eggs in a small bowl with the yogurt and salt.

Heat the butter in an 8-inch oven-safe frying pan over medium heat. When the butter has melted, add the asparagus and cook until just tender, approximately 3 minutes. Add the egg mixture and tomato to the pan and stir with a spatula until just blended. Allow the eggs to set on the bottom, 1 to 1½ minutes.

Remove the pan from the heat and slip it under the broiler until the top of the frittata is just set and puffy, approximately 1 minute.

Loosen the frittata from the pan and place on a serving dish. Serve immediately.

Fresh Veggie Frittata

SERVES 2

This vegetable frittata is light and flavorful. The spinach provides many necessary nutrients, but it also contains goitrogens. Heat the spinach well to help mitigate its goitrogenic effects.

3 eggs
1 teaspoon fat-free milk
1 tablespoon olive oil
1 handful baby spinach
½ baby eggplant, peeled and diced
¼ small red bell pepper, seeded and chopped
Iodized table salt and freshly ground black pepper
1 ounce crumbled goat cheese

Preheat the broiler.

Beat the eggs with the fat-free milk in a small bowl until just combined.

Heat a small nonstick, oven-safe skillet over medium-high heat. Add the olive oil, followed by the egg mixture. Spread the spinach on top of the egg mixture in an even layer and top with the eggplant and red bell pepper. Reduce the heat to medium and season with salt and pepper.

Allow the eggs and vegetables to cook until the underside of the eggs is firm and the vegetables are tender, 3 to 5 minutes. Top with the crumbled goat cheese.

Place the pan under the broiler. Cook until the eggs are firm in the middle and the cheese has melted, 3 to 5 minutes.

Loosen the frittata from the skillet, place on a serving dish, and cut in half. Serve immediately.

Tuna-Tomato Frittata

SERVES 4

Tuna provides much-needed iodine to those people with hypothyroidism who are iodine deficient. Tomatoes also assist thyroid functioning by contributing selenium.

6 eggs, beaten
Two 5-ounce cans tuna packed in oil, drained
¼ cup fat-free milk
3 tablespoons chopped fresh flat-leaf parsley
½ teaspoon iodized table salt, plus more to taste
½ teaspoon freshly ground black pepper
1 tablespoon olive oil
1 tablespoon unsalted butter
2 tomatoes, seeded and chopped
1 cup ricotta cheese
Juice of 1 lemon

Preheat the oven to 400°F.

Mix together the eggs, tuna, milk, parsley, ½ teaspoon of the salt, and the pepper in a large bowl.

Heat the oil and butter in a 10-inch nonstick, oven-safe skillet over medium-high heat. Add the egg mixture and cook without stirring for 5 minutes.

Place the tomatoes on top of the egg mixture and continue cooking for 3 minutes.

Place the skillet in the oven and bake until the center is set, 7 to 8 minutes.

Meanwhile, in a small bowl, mix the ricotta cheese with the lemon juice.

When the frittata is ready, loosen it from the skillet, place on a serving plate, season with salt and cut into four wedges. Serve each wedge topped with a spoonful of the cheese mixture.

Mediterranean Scrambled Eggs with Garlic and Basil

SERVES 2

Eggs are a great source of protein, and with basil and garlic adding Mediterranean flavor, this breakfast staple is anything but bland. Serve this dish with fruit for a well-rounded meal.

4 eggs

2 tablespoons finely chopped fresh basil

2 tablespoons grated Gruyère cheese

1 tablespoon heavy cream

1 tablespoon olive oil

2 garlic cloves, minced

Iodized table salt and freshly ground black pepper

In a large bowl, beat together the eggs, basil, cheese, and cream with a whisk until just combined.

Heat the oil in a large, nonstick skillet over medium-low heat. Add the garlic and cook until golden, about 1 minute. Pour the egg mixture over the garlic. Work the eggs continuously and cook until fluffy and soft, 3 to 5 minutes.

Season with salt and pepper. Divide between two plates and serve immediately.

Greek Eggs and Potatoes

Load these eggs with fresh tomatoes, garlic, and herbs for a boost of nutrition and flavor. For extra texture and fiber, leave the potato skins on the potatoes. This dish is popular when served family-style at the table.

3 medium tomatoes, seeded and coarsely chopped
2 tablespoons chopped fresh basil
1 garlic clove, minced
2 tablespoons plus ½ cup olive oil
Iodized table salt and freshly ground black pepper
3 large russet potatoes, diced
4 eggs
1 teaspoon chopped fresh oregano

Put the tomatoes in a food processor and purée them, skins and all. Add the basil, garlic, and 2 tablespoons of the olive oil, season with salt and pepper, and pulse to combine.

Transfer the mixture to a large skillet, cover, and cook over medium heat until the sauce has thickened and is bubbly, 15 to 20 minutes.

Meanwhile, pour the remaining ½ cup olive oil into a nonstick skillet and heat over medium-low heat. Add the potatoes and fry them until crisp and browned, about 5 minutes. Cover and reduce the heat to low. Steam until the potatoes are tender, about 7 minutes.

Carefully crack each egg into the tomato sauce. Cook over low heat until the eggs are set in the sauce, about 6 minutes.

Remove the potatoes from the pan and drain them on paper towels, then place them on a plate. Season with salt and pepper and top with oregano.

Carefully remove the eggs with a slotted spoon and place them on a plate with the potatoes. Spoon the sauce over the top and serve.

Spicy Scrambled Eggs

SERVES 4

You can enjoy whole eggs up to four times a week as part of a balanced diet. If you can stand the heat, spicy additions like jalapeño peppers not only add flavor but also help you feel full faster. Enjoy this dish with whole-wheat toast.

2 tablespoons olive oil

1 small red onion, chopped

1 medium green bell pepper, seeded and finely chopped

1 jalapeño pepper, seeded and cut into thin strips

3 medium tomatoes, chopped

Iodized table salt and freshly ground black pepper

1 tablespoon ground cumin

1 tablespoon ground coriander

4 eggs, lightly beaten

Heat the olive oil in a large skillet over medium heat. Add the onion and cook until soft and translucent, 6 to 7 minutes. Add the peppers and continue to cook until soft, another 4 to 5 minutes. Add the tomatoes and season with salt and pepper. Stir in the cumin and coriander, reduce the heat to medium-low, and simmer for 10 minutes.

Add the eggs, stirring them into the mixture to distribute. Cover the skillet and cook until the eggs are set but still fluffy and tender, 5 to 6 minutes.

Divide between 4 plates and serve immediately.

Smoked Salmon Cucumber Rolls with Dill Sauce

This dish provides the iodine and omega-3 acids that you need in a light and refreshing breakfast option. Cucumbers have antioxidants as well as anti-inflammatory properties, making them a pleasant addition to your morning meal. The dill sauce may be prepared the night before, making assembly a breeze in the morning.

Handful fresh dill
1 cup plain nonfat yogurt
8 ounces smoked salmon
1 English cucumber, cut lengthwise into 6 thin slices

Process the dill and yogurt in a blender at high speed.

Place the salmon on the cucumber slices, roll them up, and skewer them closed with toothpicks.

Serve with the dill sauce.

Poached Egg and Toast

SERVES 1

Eggs are a great source of protein, and whole-grain toast provides a good amount of fiber and a nice texture to stand up to the egg yolk.

2 tablespoons distilled white vinegar
1 egg
1 slice whole-grain toast
Iodized table salt and freshly ground black pepper

Bring a small saucepan of water, 3 inches deep, to a very low simmer over medium heat. Add the vinegar.

Break the egg into a small bowl. Pour the egg into the water and poach, about 3 to 4 minutes, occasionally nudging it with a spatula so that it stays together and does not stick to the bottom. Remove with a slotted spoon.

Serve the egg over toast, seasoned with salt and pepper.

Poached Eggs with Artichoke Hearts

SERVES 4

With artichoke hearts and mustard sauce, this Italian recipe makes poached eggs a far more interesting way to start the day. Artichoke hearts are packed with antioxidants, which help prevent heart disease.

3 tablespoons butter
1 teaspoon Dijon mustard
1 teaspoon all-purpose flour
1 cup water
2 tablespoons white wine vinegar
Iodized table salt and freshly black ground pepper
4 canned artichoke hearts, drained
2 tablespoons distilled white vinegar
4 eggs

Melt the butter in a small pan over medium heat and stir in the mustard and flour. Gradually stir in the water and white wine vinegar, alternating between the two. Stir constantly for 5 minutes. Season with salt and pepper. Reduce the heat to low.

Bring a medium saucepan of water to a boil over high heat. Add the artichoke hearts and blanch them for 3 minutes. Transfer them to a colander to drain and slice each into eight rounds. Arrange the artichokes in a ring on a serving dish.

Refill the saucepan with 3 inches of water and bring to a very low simmer over medium heat. Add the distilled white vinegar.

Break the eggs into four separate small bowls. Pour the eggs individually into the water and poach, about 3 to 4 minutes, occasionally nudging them with a spatula so that they stay together and do not stick to each other or to the bottom. Remove them with a slotted spoon.

Place the poached eggs on top of the artichokes. Spoon the mustard sauce over the artichokes and eggs and serve.

Italian Eggs with Tomatoes

SERVES 2

Simplicity is a theme in Italian cooking. With just eggs, tomatoes, and a few herbs, you have an elegant breakfast, rich in flavors. This meal provides both protein from the eggs and selenium from the tomatoes, among many of the nutritional benefits.

2 teaspoons olive oil
2 large tomatoes
Iodized table salt
Pinch of dried oregano
Freshly ground black pepper
2 eggs
Chopped fresh flat-leaf parsley, for garnish

Preheat the oven to 350°F. Brush a small baking dish with 1 teaspoon of the olive oil.

Cut off the tops of the tomatoes and scoop out the seeds and most of the flesh. Season the insides of the tomatoes with salt and place them upside down on paper towels for 10 minutes to drain.

Flip the tomatoes back up, place inside the oiled dish, and season the insides with oregano, pepper, and the remaining 1 teaspoon olive oil. Bake the tomatoes for 20 minutes.

Remove the pan from the oven and break an egg into each tomato. Return the dish to the oven and bake for an additional 5 minutes.

Garnish with parsley and serve.

Egg Muffins "On the Go"

SERVES 12

Everyone knows that eggs are a fantastic source of protein, but sometimes it is difficult to fit in a hot breakfast in the morning. These muffins can be made in advance and stored in the refrigerator, then popped in the microwave when you're ready to eat. This version includes peppers and tomatoes to boost the nutrition, and the scallions add depth to the flavor.

1 red bell pepper, seeded and chopped
2 tomatoes, chopped
3 scallions, chopped
12 eggs, beaten

Preheat the oven to 375°F.

Combine the pepper, tomatoes, and scallions in a large bowl.

Line two 12-cup mini muffin pans with cupcake liners. Fill each cup with 1 tablespoon of beaten egg. Fill the rest of each cup with the chopped vegetables.

Bake until firm on top, 15 to 20 minutes.

Serve immediately, or allow to cool and then wrap each individually and store in the refrigerator for up to 1 week. To reheat, unwrap and place in the microwave for 30 seconds.

Breakfast

Eggs with Asparagus Soldiers

SERVES 4

This dish is a cute way to enjoy soft-boiled eggs. Many children enjoy dipping their asparagus "soldiers" into the runny yolk of a soft-boiled egg. This dish is especially fun if you have egg stands or cups.

16 asparagus spears
4 eggs
8 toasted baguette slices (optional)
Iodized table salt and freshly ground black pepper

Bring a large pot of water to a boil over high heat. Trim the woody ends off the asparagus and cook until tender, about 7 minutes.

While the asparagus are cooking, bring a medium saucepan of water, 3 inches deep, to a boil over high heat. Add the eggs and cook for 4 to 5 minutes, so that the eggs are soft-boiled. Drain the hot water and add cold water to stop the eggs from cooking further.

Drain the asparagus and place under cold running water for a few seconds to stop the cooking.

Set each egg in an egg stand and "behead" it by peeling and cutting off the top of the egg shell. Serve each egg with 4 asparagus spears and toasted baguette slices, if desired. Season the eggs and asparagus with salt and pepper. To eat, dip the asparagus in the runny egg yolk.

Savory Breakfast Quinoa

SERVES 2

Savory hot cereal is not common in the United States, but it is a great way to shake things up at breakfast. This dish combines the fiber of quinoa with a mixture of tomato and cucumber, a pairing that is common in Turkey, Greece, and Israel. Meanwhile, the herbs and pepper add a little kick.

½ cup quinoa, rinsed twice and drained
1 cup water
1 large tomato, chopped
1 medium cucumber, chopped
1 tablespoon olive oil
Freshly grated, low-fat Parmesan cheese
Chopped fresh flat-leaf parsley or mint, for garnish
Iodized table salt and freshly ground black pepper

Place the quinoa and water in a medium saucepan and bring to a boil over high heat. Cover, reduce the heat to low, and simmer until the water is absorbed, about 15 minutes.

Divide the quinoa between two bowls and add the tomato and cucumber. Drizzle with olive oil, then top with the Parmesan cheese and parsley or mint. Season with salt and pepper.

Serve immediately.

Breakfast

Cinnamon Quinoa with Blueberries

SERVES 2

Packed with essential amino acids, quinoa is the perfect way to start the day. Quinoa serves as a great substitute for wheat or barley, especially for those who are gluten-intolerant. Blueberries' ability to reduce symptoms of hypothyroidism makes them a great addition to this breakfast.

½ cup quinoa, rinsed twice and drained
1 cup water
Pinch of iodized table salt
½ cup fat-free milk
1 teaspoon pure vanilla extract
¼ teaspoon ground cinnamon
1 cup fresh blueberries

48

Place the quinoa, water, and salt in a medium saucepan and bring to a boil over high heat. Cover, reduce the heat to low, and simmer until the water is absorbed, about 15 minutes.

Take the quinoa off the heat and let it stand, covered, for 5 minutes. Stir in the milk, vanilla extract, and cinnamon until fully incorporated.

Divide between two bowls, top with the berries, and serve.

Mung Bean Porridge

SERVES 6

Mung beans are commonly eaten for breakfast in Southeast Asia. They are a great source of protein and fiber, so they are very popular with vegetarians. Mung beans are good for digestion and will keep you satiated for several hours, making them a great choice for breakfast.

1 cup mung beans, rinsed
4½ cups water
1 cinnamon stick
¼ teaspoon iodized table salt
1 teaspoon pure vanilla extract
1 cup unsweetened coconut milk

Place the mung beans, water, and cinnamon in a large saucepan and bring to a boil over high heat. Reduce the heat to low and simmer until the beans have cracked but are not mushy, about 40 minutes.

Add the salt and vanilla extract. Stir in the coconut milk until heated through, about 2 minutes.

Remove the cinnamon stick. Ladle the porridge into bowls. Serve warm.

Healthier Banana Bread

YIELDS 1 LOAF

This banana bread has been revamped from the traditional version. Instead of regular flour, this banana bread uses quinoa flour, which is high in protein. The recipe calls for maple syrup and honey as opposed to processed sugar, creating a more complex flavor and making use of more natural ingredients.

1 egg
¼ cup pure maple syrup
¼ cup honey
¼ teaspoon coconut oil, plus more to grease the pan
1½ cups quinoa flour, plus more for sprinkling the pan
4 very ripe bananas
1 teaspoon baking soda
1 teaspoon baking powder
¼ teaspoon iodized table salt

Preheat the oven to 350°F.

Combine the egg, maple syrup, honey, and ¼ teaspoon of the coconut oil in a large bowl. Add the bananas, baking soda, baking powder, and salt and mix with an electric mixer.

Grease a 9-by-5-inch loaf pan with a little coconut oil and sprinkle with quinoa flour to prevent the banana bread from sticking. Pour the batter into the pan.

Bake for 45 minutes.

Let cool slightly, slice, and serve.

Baked Berry Oatmeal

SERVES 6

Whole grains such as oats provide a substantial amount of vitamin B as well as selenium. They also help alleviate constipation, which is a common complaint among those who suffer from hypothyroidism. Brazil nuts are helpful to the thyroid, but if Brazil nut milk makes this recipe too nutty for you, feel free to substitute regular fat-free milk. (Make sure to allow time in between taking thyroid medication and consuming walnuts, as they interfere with certain medications.)

2 cups rolled oats

½ cup chopped walnuts, toasted

1½ teaspoons ground cinnamon

1 teaspoon baking powder

½ teaspoon iodized table salt

2 cups Brazil Nut Milk (see p. 52) or fat-free milk

1 egg

⅓ cup maple syrup

3 tablespoons unsalted butter, melted

2 teaspoons pure vanilla extract

2 bananas, sliced (½ inch thick)

1½ cups fresh or frozen blueberries

Preheat the oven to 375°F. Coat the inside of an 8-inch square baking dish with cooking spray.

In a medium bowl, combine the oats, half of the walnuts, the cinnamon, baking powder, and salt.

In another medium bowl, whisk together the milk, egg, syrup, half of the butter, and the vanilla.

Spread a single layer of bananas across the bottom of the baking dish. Sprinkle two-thirds of the blueberries on top. Cover with the oat mixture, then drizzle the milk mixture over the oats. Top with the remaining blueberries and walnuts.

Bake until golden brown, 35 to 45 minutes.

Cool for a few minutes. Drizzle the remaining butter on top and serve.

Breakfast

Brazil Nut Milk

YIELDS ABOUT 7 CUPS

Brazil nuts are a fantastic natural source of healthy fats as well as selenium, a trace mineral that is necessary for proper thyroid function. Brazil nut milk, much like dairy milk, may be used in smoothies, with cereal, or simply poured over ice.

4 cups raw Brazil nuts
6 cups water
1 tablespoon honey
2 teaspoons pure vanilla extract

Place the Brazil nuts in a bowl and cover with the water. Soak for 8 hours.

Place the nuts and water in a blender and blend on high speed until smooth-ish, about 1 minute.

Pour the nut milk through a cheesecloth-lined strainer, then return to the blender. Add the honey and vanilla and blend until well combined.

Store in the refrigerator for up to 5 days.

Brazil Nut and Banana Breakfast Smoothie

This quick smoothie is full of protein and rich in selenium. Brazil nuts are gaining in popularity because of their high content of selenium as well as healthy fats.

1 cup Brazil Nut Milk (see facing page)
1 frozen banana
2 tablespoons unsweetened cocoa powder

Place all the ingredients in a blender and blend until smooth. Serve.

Quick Chocolate-Banana Smoothie

SERVES 1

This breakfast smoothie resembles a chocolate milk shake and is sure to please adults and children alike. Bananas provide potassium that heals muscles, making this a perfect breakfast before or after a morning workout. The Brazil Nut Milk gives the smoothie a subtle nutty flavor as well as selenium.

1 ripe banana
½ cup Brazil Nut Milk (see p. 52)
2 tablespoons unsweetened cocoa powder
3 or 4 ice cubes

Place all the ingredients in a blender and blend until smooth (it will not be as thick as a typical smoothie). Serve.

Power-Packed
Banana-Quinoa Smoothie

SERVES 1

This smoothie is packed with good nutrients, and it's a good use for leftover plain quinoa. (Make sure to allow time in between taking thyroid medication and consuming walnuts, as they interfere with certain medications.)

1 cup water
1 frozen banana
⅓ cup cooked quinoa
1 tablespoon honey
1 teaspoon ground cinnamon
½ teaspoon pure vanilla extract
1 tablespoon chopped raw walnuts, for topping (optional)

Place all the ingredients except the walnuts in a blender and blend until smooth, about 1 minute. Pour into a glass and top with chopped walnuts, if desired, and serve.

Super Avocado and Honey Smoothie

Known as a "superfood," avocados are loaded with heart-healthy monounsaturated fats. This quick and simple smoothie is a great breakfast on the go. Loaded with fiber, it will definitely fill you up in the morning.

1½ cups fat-free milk
1 large avocado, pitted and peeled
2 tablespoons honey

Place all the ingredients in a blender and blend until smooth and creamy. Pour into two glasses and serve.

Blueberry-Banana Smoothie

Smoothies are a great way to pack nutrients into breakfast. Loaded with antioxidants, blueberries boost immunity. Bananas' fiber content helps to stave off hunger until lunch.

½ medium banana
1 cup frozen blueberries
½ cup nonfat yogurt
½ cup fat-free milk
½ cup ice

Place all the ingredients in a blender and blend until smooth. Pour into two glasses and serve.

Blueberry-Avocado Smoothie

SERVES 1

This smoothie features two fruits commonly believed to be "superfoods" because of their high nutritional content. The antioxidants from blueberries and healthy fats from the avocado make this a well-rounded meal. Including the protein from Greek yogurt, this smoothie covers almost all your nutritional bases.

1 cup nonfat Greek yogurt
1 cup frozen blueberries
½ avocado, pitted and peeled
¼ cup low-fat milk

Combine all the ingredients in a blender and blend until smooth. Serve.

Blueberry-Cherry Parfait

SERVES 1

A parfait is a simple and elegant dish that may be served as breakfast or dessert. The concept is very versatile, and you should feel free to use whatever fruit you prefer. This recipe takes advantage of blueberries and cherries, both rich in disease-fighting antioxidants.

1½ cups nonfat plain or vanilla yogurt
½ cup fresh blueberries
½ cup fresh cherries, pitted and halved

Place ½ cup of the yogurt in a tall glass. Place half of the blueberries over the yogurt. Cover the blueberries with another ½ cup of the yogurt. Place half of the cherries over the yogurt. Add the remaining ½ cup yogurt, then the remaining blueberries and cherries. Serve.

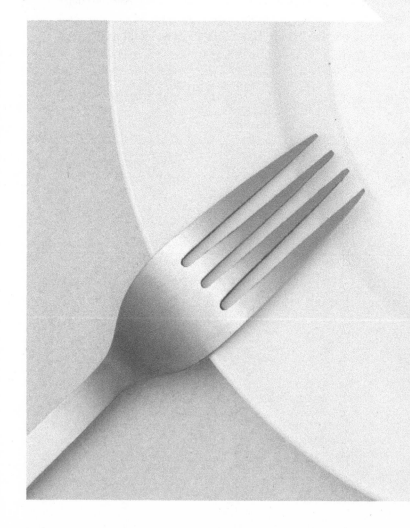

CHAPTER EIGHT

Lunch

Seaweed Salad

SERVES 2

Similar to dark leafy greens, seaweed is about as nutrient dense as it gets, packed with vitamins such as C (even more than broccoli), B$_{12}$, and A. The iodine content helps the thyroid function. As seaweed has become more popular, you can find it at most large grocery stores.

One 3-ounce package seaweed salad mix
1 tablespoon sesame seeds
4 teaspoons rice vinegar
4 teaspoons reduced-sodium soy sauce
1 teaspoon toasted sesame oil
½ teaspoon sugar
1 scallion, chopped

In a large bowl, soak the seaweed salad mix in cold water for 5 minutes or according to the package directions. Drain and transfer to a serving bowl.

Toast the sesame seeds in a dry skillet over medium heat until lightly golden.

In a small bowl, combine the rice vinegar, soy sauce, sesame oil, sugar, scallion, and toasted sesame seeds.

Pour the dressing over the seaweed and toss to thoroughly combine. Serve.

Asparagus Salad

SERVES 4

Asparagus is a spring vegetable that is delicious both raw and cooked. Asparagus is not only low in calories, but it is also a good source of vitamins B_6, calcium, magnesium, and zinc. Since it is not a cruciferous vegetable, asparagus is a good way to eat vegetables without lowering your thyroid function.

1 pound asparagus
Iodized table salt and freshly ground black pepper
¼ cup olive oil
1 tablespoon balsamic vinegar
1 tablespoon freshly grated lemon zest

Shave the asparagus with a vegetable peeler into thin strips. (Alternatively, you can roast the asparagus in a baking pan with a little of the olive oil for 15 minutes at 400°F.)

Season with salt and pepper, then toss with the olive oil and vinegar. Garnish with a sprinkle of lemon zest and serve.

Endive with Shrimp

SERVES 4

This elegant, simple salad makes a delicious entrée for a small luncheon. The walnuts provide high levels of omega-3 fatty acids. (Make sure to allow time in between taking thyroid medication and consuming walnuts, as they interfere with certain medications.) Serve this salad with a dry white wine.

½ cup olive oil
1 small shallot, minced
1 tablespoon Dijon mustard
Juice and zest of 1 lemon
Iodized table salt and freshly ground black pepper
2 cups water
14 medium shrimp, peeled and deveined
1 head endive
½ cup diced tart green apple
2 tablespoons chopped toasted walnuts

Whisk together the olive oil, shallot, mustard, and lemon juice and zest in a small bowl until creamy and emulsified. Season with salt and pepper. Cover and refrigerate for at least 2 hours for best flavor.

Fill a small pan with water and add some salt. Bring to a boil, add the shrimp, and cook until the shrimp turn pink, 1 to 2 minutes. Drain and cool under cold water.

To assemble the salad, tear the endive into bite-size pieces. Place on serving plates and top with the shrimp, green apple, and toasted walnuts. Drizzle with the vinaigrette and serve.

Lunch

Four-Bean Salad

SERVES 4

Inspired by the Mediterranean, this bean salad is both healthy and delicious. Beans are high in fiber, keeping you satiated until dinner. Use dried beans for the best flavor (you can cook them a day or two in advance), but keep canned beans on hand as a convenient option.

½ cup cooked or canned white beans, rinsed and drained

½ cup cooked or canned black-eyed peas, rinsed and drained

½ cup cooked or canned fava beans, rinsed and drained

½ cup cooked or canned lima beans, rinsed and drained

1 red bell pepper, seeded and diced

1 small bunch fresh flat-leaf parsley, chopped

2 tablespoons olive oil

1 teaspoon ground cumin

Juice of 1 lemon

Iodized table salt and freshly ground black pepper

Combine all the ingredients except the salt and pepper in a large bowl and mix well. Season with salt and pepper.

Allow the salad to sit for 30 minutes at room temperature so the flavors can come together. Serve.

Garden Salad with Sardine Fillets

SERVES 4

Sardines are nutrition dense, containing vitamins B$_3$, B$_{12}$, and D, as well as tryptophan, selenium, omega-3 fats, protein, phosphorus, and calcium. In this recipe, sardines turn a simple garden salad into a filling lunch.

½ cup olive oil
Juice of 1 lemon
1 teaspoon Dijon mustard
Iodized table salt and freshly ground black pepper
4 medium tomatoes, diced
1 large cucumber, peeled and diced
1 pound arugula, trimmed and chopped
1 small red onion, thinly sliced
1 small bunch fresh flat-leaf parsley, chopped
4 whole sardine fillets packed in olive oil, drained and chopped

Whisk together the olive oil, lemon juice, and mustard, and season with salt and pepper. Set aside.

In a large bowl, combine the tomatoes, cucumber, arugula, onion, and parsley, and toss. Add the sardine fillets on top of the salad.

Drizzle the dressing over the salad just before serving.

Moroccan Tomato and Roasted Pepper Salad with Grilled Chicken

SERVES 6

This dish features plenty of vegetables that one finds in the Mediterranean, served with grilled chicken.

2 large green bell peppers, halved lengthwise and seeded

1 jalapeño pepper, halved lengthwise and seeded

4 large tomatoes, peeled, seeded, and diced

1 small bunch fresh flat-leaf parsley, chopped

¼ cup olive oil

1 teaspoon ground cumin

Juice of 1 lemon

Iodized table salt and freshly ground black pepper

6 grilled chicken breasts

Preheat the broiler. Place the bell peppers and jalapeño pepper on a baking sheet, cut-sides down. Broil until the skins blacken and blister, 5 to 10 minutes. Transfer the peppers to a paper bag. Seal and set aside to cool.

Combine the tomatoes, parsley, olive oil, cumin, and lemon juice in a medium bowl and mix well.

Take the peppers out of the bag and peel off the skins under running water, then pat dry with paper towels. Chop the peppers and add them to the salad. Season with salt and pepper. Toss to combine and let the salad sit at room temperature for 15 to 20 minutes.

To serve, divide the salad among six plates and place a chicken breast over each portion.

Raw Zucchini Salad

SERVES 2

This healthy salad makes an excellent light lunch. Zucchini and tomatoes are especially flavorful in the summer and provide good nutrition. The key to this dish's success is to slice the zucchini paper-thin with a mandoline or vegetable peeler, or shred it into long, thin ribbons with a cheese grater. Since this salad is low calorie, feel free to go for seconds!

1 medium zucchini, shredded or sliced paper thin

6 cherry tomatoes, halved

3 tablespoons olive oil

Juice of 1 lemon

Iodized table salt and freshly ground black pepper

3 or 4 leaves fresh basil, thinly sliced

2 tablespoons freshly grated low-fat Parmesan cheese

Layer the zucchini slices evenly on two plates. Top with the tomatoes. Drizzle with the olive oil and lemon juice. Season with salt and pepper. Top with the basil and sprinkle with cheese before serving.

Cold Cucumber Soup

SERVES 4

Take advantage of this refreshing soup on a hot summer's day. Serve it with pita bread or a salad for a light lunch or dinner. Feel free to substitute regular nonfat yogurt for Greek yogurt.

2 English cucumbers, peeled and cut into chunks
2 cups plain Greek yogurt
½ cup finely chopped fresh mint
2 garlic cloves, minced
2 cups reduced-sodium vegetable broth
1 tablespoon chopped fresh dill
1 tablespoon tomato paste
Iodized table salt and freshly ground black pepper

Purée the cucumbers, yogurt, mint, and garlic in a food processor or blender. Add the vegetable broth, dill, and tomato paste and blend completely. Season with salt and pepper.

Refrigerate for at least 2 hours before serving.

Italian Cream of Mushroom Soup with Red Wine

SERVES 6

The classic flavors of Italy—red wine and mushrooms—are combined in this rich and creamy soup. Mushrooms are a good source of vitamins B_2, B_3, and B_5, as well as selenium. Substitute cremini or oyster mushrooms for the button mushrooms, if you prefer.

2 ounces dried porcini
2 ounces dried morels
1 tablespoon olive oil
1 teaspoon butter
8 ounces portobello mushrooms, chopped
8 ounces button mushrooms, chopped
3 shallots, finely chopped
2 garlic cloves, minced
1 teaspoon finely chopped fresh thyme
Iodized table salt and freshly ground black pepper
4 cups reduced-sodium chicken broth
⅓ cup dry red wine or sherry
½ cup heavy cream
1 small bunch flat-leaf parsley, chopped, for garnish

Reconstitute the dried mushrooms by pouring enough warm water over them to cover and allowing them to sit for 30 minutes. Drain, chop, and set aside.

In a large Dutch oven or stockpot, heat the olive oil and butter over medium-high heat. Add the reconstituted and fresh mushrooms and the shallots, and cook until the mushrooms are softened, about 10 minutes. Add the garlic and cook for 1 minute more. Add the thyme, and season with salt and pepper.

Add the broth and wine, increase the heat to high, and bring to a boil. Reduce the heat to low and simmer for 20 minutes.

Remove half of the soup, purée it in a food processor or blender, then add it back to the pot. This will thicken the soup while still leaving some of the mushrooms intact for textural contrast. (Alternatively, you can use a handheld immersion blender to purée some of the soup right in the pot.)

Stir in the cream and warm through. Ladle into bowls, garnish with the parsley, and serve.

Farro Bean Soup

This comforting soup is inexpensive, highly nutritious, and easy to make. Farro is a rustic grain that you can find at health food stores if your grocer doesn't carry it.

2 tablespoons olive oil

1 medium onion, diced

1 celery rib, diced

2 garlic cloves, minced

8 cups reduced-sodium chicken broth or water

1 cup dried white beans, soaked overnight, rinsed, and drained

One 14½-ounce can diced tomatoes, undrained

1 cup farro

½ teaspoon dried thyme

½ teaspoon freshly ground black pepper, plus more for seasoning

2 bay leaves

Iodized table salt

Heat the olive oil in a large Dutch oven or stockpot over medium-high heat. Sauté the onion, celery, and garlic just until tender, about 5 minutes.

Add the broth or water, beans, tomatoes with their juice, farro, thyme, pepper, and bay leaves, and bring to a simmer. Reduce heat, cover, and cook until the beans and farro are tender, about 2 hours. Remove the bay leaves.

Season with salt and pepper and serve.

Roasted Eggplant Soup

SERVES 8

Soup is a wonderful option for a healthy lunch. Fresh herbs add flavor to this soup as well as powerful nutrients and antioxidants. This soup is best served with bread.

Iodized table salt
3 large eggplants, halved lengthwise
2 tablespoons olive oil
1 medium red onion, chopped
2 tablespoons minced garlic
1 teaspoon dried thyme
Freshly ground black pepper
2 large tomatoes, halved
5 cups reduced-sodium chicken broth
¼ cup light cream
1 small bunch fresh mint, chopped, for garnish

Preheat the oven to 400°F.

Lightly salt both sides of the eggplant halves; and let sit in a colander in the sink for 20 minutes to draw out the bitter juices. Rinse the eggplants and pat dry with a paper towel.

Place the eggplants on a baking sheet and put them in the oven to roast for 45 minutes.

Remove the eggplants from the oven and allow to cool, then remove all the flesh, discarding the skins.

Heat the olive oil in a large skillet over medium heat. Add the onion and garlic and cook until soft and translucent, about 5 minutes. Add the thyme and season with salt and pepper.

Put the eggplant, tomatoes, and the onion-garlic mixture in a food processor and process until smooth.

Bring the chicken broth to a boil in a large Dutch oven or stockpot over high heat. Reduce the heat to a simmer, and add the processed vegetable mixture. Stir until well combined and fold in the cream.

Season with more salt and pepper, if needed. Serve the soup garnished with the fresh mint.

Greek Roasted Red Pepper and Feta Soup

SERVES 6

A traditional combination of red peppers and feta makes this soup both sweet and savory. This Mediterranean dish also provides plenty of nutrition. Serve with crusty bread or pita.

10 red bell peppers, halved lengthwise and seeded
2 red chile peppers, halved lengthwise and seeded
2 tablespoons olive oil
1 medium red onion, chopped
4 garlic cloves, minced
2 teaspoons finely chopped fresh oregano
6 cups reduced-sodium chicken broth
Iodized table salt and freshly ground black pepper
¼ cup light cream
Juice of 1 lemon
6 tablespoons crumbled Greek feta

Preheat the broiler. Place the bell peppers and chile peppers on a baking sheet, cut-sides down. Broil until the skins blacken and blister, 5 to 10 minutes. Transfer the peppers to a paper bag. Seal and set aside to cool.

When cool, take the peppers out of the bag and peel off the skins under running water, them pat them dry with a paper towel. Put the roasted peppers in a food processor and process until smooth.

Heat the olive oil in a large Dutch oven or stockpot over medium-high heat and add the onion and garlic. Cook until soft and translucent, about 5 minutes. Add the pepper mixture and oregano, followed by the broth. Increase the heat to high and bring to a boil. Season with salt and pepper, reduce the heat to low, and simmer for 15 minutes.

Stir in the cream and lemon juice.

Ladle into bowls, top with the crumbled feta, and serve immediately.

Provençal Shrimp Soup with Leeks and Fennel

SERVES 6

The Provençal flavors of leeks, fennel, garlic, and shrimp are featured in this elegant soup. Seafood is a great source of iodine, which helps the thyroid function properly. Scallops also work well in this dish.

2 tablespoons olive oil
3 celery ribs, chopped
1 leek, white and light green parts, sliced
1 medium fennel bulb, chopped
1 garlic clove, minced
Iodized table salt and freshly ground black pepper
1 tablespoon fennel seeds
4 cups reduced-sodium vegetable broth
1 pound medium shrimp, peeled and deveined
2 tablespoons light cream
Juice of 1 lemon

Heat the oil in a large Dutch oven or stockpot over medium heat. Add the celery, leek, and fennel and cook until the vegetables are browned and very soft, about 15 minutes.

Add the garlic and season with salt and pepper. Stir in the fennel seeds.

Add the broth and bring to boil, then reduce to a simmer and cook for 20 more minutes.

Add the shrimp to the soup and cook until just pink, about 3 minutes.

Stir in the cream and lemon juice. Serve immediately.

Moroccan Tomato Soup

SERVES 6

Not your everyday tomato soup, this one is subtly flavored with the classic spices of Morocco—paprika, ginger, cumin, and cinnamon. In terms of nutrients, cooked tomatoes are a great source of lycopene. Enjoy this soup with a side of bread.

2 tablespoons olive oil

1 large onion, coarsely chopped

8 large tomatoes, seeded and coarsely chopped

1 teaspoon paprika

1 teaspoon finely chopped fresh ginger

1 teaspoon ground cumin

2 cups reduced-sodium chicken broth

1 cinnamon stick

1 teaspoon honey

Iodized table salt and freshly ground black pepper

Juice of 1 lemon

2 tablespoons chopped fresh flat-leaf parsley, for garnish

2 tablespoons chopped fresh cilantro, for garnish

Heat the oil in a large Dutch oven or stockpot over medium-high heat. Add the onion and cook until soft and translucent, about 5 minutes. Stir in the tomatoes, paprika, ginger, and cumin.

Pour in the chicken broth, add the cinnamon stick and honey, lower the heat, and simmer for 15 minutes. Remove the cinnamon stick and transfer the soup to a food processor or blender. Purée the soup until smooth. Pour it back into the pot and reheat, then season with salt and pepper.

Stir in the lemon juice and serve, garnished with the parsley and cilantro.

Turkish Lentil Soup

SERVES 6

Lentil soup is one of the most inexpensive, nutritious foods you can make. If you can't find green lentils, substitute brown. This Turkish-inspired recipe is vegetarian, but feel free to add shredded ham or chicken for a more robust dish.

2 tablespoons olive oil
1 small onion, diced
2 tablespoons flour
4 cups water or reduced-sodium chicken broth
1½ cups green lentils
1 carrot, peeled and diced
1 teaspoon iodized table salt
½ teaspoon freshly ground black pepper
½ teaspoon dried thyme

Heat the olive oil in a large Dutch oven or stockpot over medium-high heat. Sauté the onion just until tender and translucent, about 5 minutes. Whisk in the flour, stirring for 30 seconds until thickened into a paste.

Slowly whisk in the water (or chicken broth), ¼ cup at a time, and bring to a boil, stirring frequently.

Add the lentils, carrot, salt, pepper, and thyme. Lower the heat, cover, and simmer until the lentils are tender, about 1 hour. Serve.

Lunch

Zuppa di Fagioli

SERVES 8

Beans are great for lowering cholesterol. Traditionally, this Tuscan soup is made with cannellini beans or cranberry beans, but you can use navy beans, white beans, or even chickpeas.

2 tablespoons olive oil

3 carrots, peeled and diced

1 onion, chopped

2 garlic cloves, chopped

8 cups water or reduced-sodium chicken broth

2 cups dried beans, soaked overnight, rinsed, and drained

1 teaspoon chopped fresh thyme

1 bay leaf

Iodized table salt and freshly ground black pepper

8 slices whole-wheat bread

Freshly grated low-fat Parmesan cheese

Heat the olive oil in a large Dutch oven or stockpot over medium heat. Add the carrots and onion and sauté until the onion is translucent, about 5 minutes. Add the garlic and sauté for 1 minute more.

Add the water (or chicken broth), beans, thyme, and bay leaf, and cover. Increase the heat to high and bring to a boil, then lower the heat and simmer, covered, until the beans are tender, about 2 hours. Remove the bay leaf.

Season with salt and pepper and ladle out the soup, topping each serving with a slice of toasted whole-wheat bread and some grated Parmesan cheese.

Korean Seaweed Soup

SERVES 4

Known as miyeok guk, this is an everyday food for Koreans but is also served on birthdays and for new moms after childbirth. Wakame (brown seaweed) is rich in minerals and high in iron and potassium. Recently, seaweed has gained popularity and is available in many supermarkets.

1 ounce dried seaweed (wakame)
2 tablespoons toasted sesame oil
¼ pound beef top sirloin, chopped
2 tablespoons reduced-sodium soy sauce
Iodized table salt
6 cups water

Soak the dried seaweed in enough water to cover it until soft and fully rehydrated, 30 to 40 minutes. Drain the seaweed and cut into bite-size pieces.

Heat the sesame oil in a large Dutch oven or stockpot over medium heat. Add the beef, 1 tablespoon of the soy sauce, and a pinch of salt. Cook for 1 minute.

Add the seaweed and the remaining 1 tablespoon soy sauce to the pot. Cook for 1 minute, stirring frequently.

Pour the water into the pot. Increase the heat to high and bring to a boil. Cover, reduce the heat, and simmer for 20 minutes.

Season with more salt if desired and serve.

Mediterranean Tuna Salad Sandwiches

SERVES 2

Usually loaded with high-fat mayonnaise, tuna salad does not often come to mind as a nutritious staple. This version is made with Greek yogurt and flavorful roasted peppers, adding taste and moisture without a lot of fat. You can also enjoy the tuna salad without the bread, over salad greens, if you prefer.

One 5-ounce can white tuna, packed in water or olive oil, drained
1 roasted red bell pepper, diced
½ small red onion, diced
10 olives, pitted and finely chopped
¼ cup plain Greek yogurt
1 tablespoon chopped fresh flat-leaf parsley
Juice of 1 lemon
Iodized table salt and freshly ground black pepper
4 slices whole-grain bread, toasted

In a small bowl, combine the tuna, bell pepper, onion, olives, yogurt, parsley, and lemon juice; mix well. Season with salt and pepper.

Spoon the tuna salad onto two pieces of toast, top with the remaining two pieces of toast to make sandwiches, and serve.

Open-Faced Eggplant Parmesan Sandwiches

SERVES 2

This recipe will help you accomplish the impossible—make healthy eggplant Parmesan sandwiches. The eggplant is broiled before being topped with marinara sauce and low-fat Parmesan cheese, and served on a slice of toasted whole-grain bread. Eat with a knife and fork!

Iodized table salt
1 small eggplant, sliced crosswise into ¼-inch rounds
2 tablespoons olive oil
Freshly ground pepper
2 thick slices whole-grain bread, toasted
1 cup marinara sauce (no added sugar)
¼ cup freshly grated low-fat Parmesan cheese

Preheat the broiler.

Lightly salt the eggplant rounds on both sides and let sit in a colander in the sink for 20 minutes to draw out the bitter juices. Rinse the eggplant slices, pat dry with a paper towel, and place on a baking sheet. Brush the eggplant slices with the olive oil and season with salt and pepper. Broil until crisp, about 4 minutes. Flip over and crisp the other side.

Lay the toasted bread slices on the baking sheet. Spoon half of the marinara sauce over the bread and layer the eggplant slices on top. Sprinkle on half of the cheese, add the rest of the marinara sauce, then sprinkle with the remaining cheese.

Put the sandwiches under the broiler until the cheese has melted, about 2 minutes.

Using a spatula, transfer the sandwiches to plates and serve.

Open-Faced Grilled Caesar Salad Sandwiches

SERVES 2

Caesar salad remains one of the most popular salads to date. This salad is an updated version of the classic. Although this salad includes a hearty amount of olive oil, this type of oil provides good fat that lowers cholesterol.

2 romaine hearts, left intact
¾ cup olive oil
3 or 4 anchovy fillets
Juice of 1 lemon
2 or 3 garlic cloves, peeled
1 teaspoon Dijon mustard
¼ teaspoon Worcestershire sauce
Iodized table salt and freshly ground black pepper
2 thick slices whole-wheat bread, toasted
Freshly grated low-fat Parmesan cheese

Heat a grill over medium-high heat. Oil the grates.

On a cutting board, drizzle the romaine hearts with 1 to 2 tablespoons of the olive oil and place them on the grates. Grill for 5 minutes, turning, until the lettuce is slightly charred on all sides.

Set the lettuce aside until it is cool enough to handle.

Meanwhile, in a food processor, combine the remaining olive oil with the anchovies, lemon juice, garlic, mustard, and Worcestershire sauce. Pulse until you have a smooth emulsion. Season with salt and pepper.

Cut the grilled lettuce in half lengthwise and place on the toasted bread.

Drizzle with the dressing and top with the Parmesan cheese. Serve.

Caprese Panini

SERVES 2

Inspired by the popular Italian caprese salad, this sandwich features tomatoes and mozzarella. Unlike the traditional caprese salad, the tomatoes are slowly roasted, which not only intensifies the flavor but increases their lycopene. If you don't have a panini maker or grill pan, you can easily toast the sandwich in a nonstick skillet.

4 Roma tomatoes, halved

4 garlic cloves

2 tablespoons olive oil

1 tablespoon dried Italian seasoning blend

Iodized table salt and freshly ground black pepper

4 leaves fresh basil

2 slices fresh mozzarella

4 slices whole-grain bread

Preheat the oven to 250°F.

Lay the tomatoes, cut-sides up, and the garlic cloves on a baking sheet, and drizzle with the olive oil. Sprinkle with Italian seasoning and season with the salt and pepper. Roast until the tomatoes are extremely fragrant and slightly wilted, 2 ½ to 3 hours.

To make the panini layer the tomatoes and garlic with the basil and cheese on the bread.

Preheat a panini maker and cook the sandwiches until the bread is browned and the cheese is melted. (Alternatively, heat a grill pan over medium-high heat and place the sandwich directly on the grill pan. Place another pan on top to press the sandwich. Flip the panini when the bread has nice grill marks, 3 to 4 minutes, and cook the other side.)

Serve warm.

Crunchy Pea and Barley Salad

Whole grains are an important part of the Mediterranean diet. Quick-cooking barley doesn't take long to prepare and is loaded with fiber and antioxidants. This salad makes a filling vegetarian meal.

2 cups water
2 cups quick-cooking barley
2 cups sugar snap peas
Small bunch chopped fresh flat-leaf parsley
½ small red onion, diced
2 tablespoons olive oil
Juice of 1 lemon
Iodized table salt and freshly ground black pepper

Bring the water to a boil in a saucepan over high heat. Stir in the barley, cover, and reduce the heat to medium-low. Simmer until all the water is absorbed, about 10 minutes. Remove from the heat and let stand, covered, for 5 minutes.

Rinse the barley under cold water, drain, and combine it with the peas, parsley, onion, olive oil, and lemon juice. Season with salt and pepper and serve.

Southwestern Quinoa and Black Bean Salad

SERVES 2 AS A MAIN COURSE OR 4 AS AN APPETIZER

Thyroid disorders often involve gluten intolerance. Both protein rich and gluten-free, quinoa is a wonderful stand-in for pasta. Quinoa's high protein content helps normalize the thyroid function. Quinoa has a bitter coating, so rinse and drain the quinoa at least twice before using.

½ cup quinoa, rinsed twice and drained
1 teaspoon coconut oil
One 15-ounce can black beans, rinsed and drained
2 cups diced fresh tomatoes
1 cup diced yellow bell pepper
2 tablespoons chopped scallions
2 teaspoons chopped jalapeño peppers
1 tablespoon chopped fresh cilantro
1 teaspoon chopped fresh basil
¼ teaspoon ground cumin
¼ teaspoon ground coriander
1 teaspoon iodized table salt
½ teaspoon freshly ground black pepper
4 teaspoons freshly squeezed lemon juice
2 cups chopped romaine lettuce

Place the quinoa and water in a medium saucepan and bring to a boil over high heat. Cover, reduce the heat to low, and simmer until the water is absorbed, about 15 minutes. Set aside to cool slightly.

In a medium skillet, heat the coconut oil over low heat. Add the beans, tomatoes, bell pepper, scallions, jalapeños, cilantro, basil, cumin, and coriander and cook for 5 minutes.

Add the quinoa, season with salt and pepper, and stir just until warmed through. Remove from the heat and sprinkle with the lemon juice.

To serve, divide the lettuce between two plates (or four if serving as an appetizer) and spoon the warm quinoa mixture on top.

Smoky Black Bean Burgers

SERVES 4

Black beans are a great source of tyrosine, an amino acid that helps the thyroid function. Black beans tend to retain moisture better than other meat substitutes. Packed with protein and flavored with liquid smoke, these vegetarian burgers are a fantastic substitute for the typical beef fare.

1 tablespoon ground flaxseeds

3 tablespoons water

One 15-ounce can black beans, rinsed and drained

¼ cup panko bread crumbs

1 garlic clove, minced

½ teaspoon iodized table salt

½ tablespoon Worcestershire sauce

¼ teaspoon liquid smoke flavoring

2 tablespoons coconut oil

4 whole-grain rolls or lettuce leaves for serving

Whisk the flaxseeds and water together in a small bowl. Let stand for about 5 minutes, or until thickened.

Using a fork or a potato masher, mash the black beans in a medium bowl until mostly smooth but still a little chunky. Add the flaxseed mixture, panko, garlic, salt, Worcestershire, and liquid smoke and stir until well combined.

Form the mixture into four patties and chill until set, about 30 minutes.

Melt the coconut oil in a skillet over medium-high heat. Sauté the bean patties for 5 minutes on each side.

Serve on whole-grain rolls or in lettuce wraps.

Perfect Summer Ratatouille

SERVES 4

Ratatouille is a classic dish from the South of France that showcases summer vegetables. These summer vegetables are rich in vital nutrients including vitamins A and C. Ratatouille is great when served over quinoa, a thyroid-friendly grain.

½ cup coconut oil
2 medium onions, sliced into thin rings
3 garlic cloves, minced
2 medium zucchini, cubed
2 medium yellow squash, cubed
2 green bell peppers, seeded and diced
1 yellow bell pepper, seeded and diced
1 red bell pepper, seeded and diced
1 medium eggplant, cubed and salted
½ teaspoon iodized table salt
¼ teaspoon freshly ground black pepper
1 bay leaf
4 sprigs fresh thyme
4 plum tomatoes, chopped
2 tablespoons chopped fresh flat-leaf parsley

In a large Dutch oven or stockpot, heat 1½ tablespoons of the coconut oil over medium-high heat. Add the onions and garlic and sauté until soft, about 5 minutes. Remove from the heat.

In a large skillet, heat another 1½ tablespoons of the coconut oil, and sauté the zucchini in batches until lightly golden on both sides. Add the zucchini to the pot with the onions.

Sauté the bell peppers in two batches in this manner, followed by the eggplant, adding 1½ tablespoons coconut oil to the skillet with each batch. Add each sautéed vegetable to the pot as it is done.

Add the salt and pepper, the bay leaf, and thyme and cover. Bring to a simmer over medium heat and cook for 15 to 20 minutes.

Add the tomatoes and parsley to the pot and simmer for 10 to 15 minutes, stirring occasionally. Remove the bay leaf and thyme sprigs and serve.

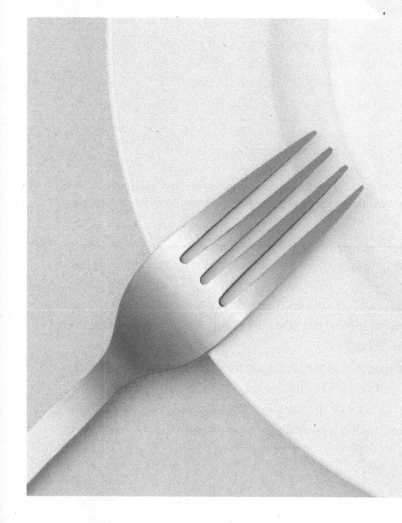

CHAPTER NINE

Dinner

Apple Couscous with Curry

SERVES 4

Couscous is a North African Berber dish, popular in Libya, Morocco, Tunisia, and Algeria. This dish has a complex variety of sweet and savory flavors. The light and fluffy couscous is stuffed with crunchy chopped pecans, but feel free to substitute walnuts or pistachios. Those who are gluten-intolerant can substitute quinoa for the couscous. (Make sure to allow time in between taking thyroid medication and consuming walnuts, as they interfere with certain medications.)

2 teaspoons olive oil
2 leeks, white parts only, sliced
1 Granny Smith apple, diced
2 cups cooked whole-wheat couscous
2 tablespoons curry powder
½ cup chopped pecans

Heat the olive oil in a large skillet over medium heat and add the leeks. Cook until soft and tender, about 5 minutes. Add the diced apple and cook until soft, about 3 minutes. Add the couscous and curry powder, then stir to combine.

Remove from the heat, stir in the nuts, and serve.

Baked Ziti

SERVES 8

Baked ziti is an American classic and the perfect dish for families or potlucks. Using whole-wheat pasta, low-fat cheese, and homemade marinara sauce makes it healthier and lighter. It can also be assembled ahead of time and baked at the last minute, and you can easily double or even triple the recipe for large groups. You will have plenty of marinara sauce left over for other uses. It will keep in a covered container in the refrigerator or in the freezer.

¼ cup olive oil
½ medium onion, diced
6 garlic cloves, minced
Two 14½-ounce cans diced tomatoes, undrained
1 sprig fresh thyme
1 bunch chopped fresh basil
Iodized table salt and freshly ground black pepper
1 pound whole-wheat ziti
1 cup low-fat cottage cheese
1 cup grated low-fat mozzarella cheese
¾ cup freshly grated low-fat Parmesan cheese

Heat the olive oil in a medium saucepan over medium-high heat. Sauté the onion and garlic, stirring until lightly browned, about 3 minutes. Add the tomatoes with their juice and the herbs and bring to a boil. Lower the heat and simmer, covered, for 10 minutes. Remove and discard the thyme sprig. Season with salt and pepper. Set the sauce aside.

Preheat the oven to 375°F.

Prepare the pasta according to the package directions. Drain and return the pasta to the pot. Add 2 cups of the marinara sauce, the cottage cheese, and half of the mozzarella and half the Parmesan and stir to combine.

Spread the mixture in a 9-by-13-inch baking dish and top with 1½ cups of the marinara sauce and the remaining cheeses.

Bake until bubbly and golden brown, 30 to 40 minutes. Serve hot.

Baked Salmon with Capers and Olives

SERVES 4

This is a fresh-tasting salmon dish inspired by the cuisine of Greece and Italy. Salmon is a great source of omega-3 fatty acids. These fatty acids help regulate the thyroid and contribute to overall good health.

1 tablespoon olive oil, divided
Four 6-ounce salmon fillets
Iodized table salt and freshly ground black pepper
2 Roma tomatoes, chopped
¼ cup pitted, chopped green olives
1 garlic clove, minced
Juice of ½ lemon
1 teaspoon capers, rinsed and drained
½ teaspoon sugar
½ cup dry bread crumbs

Preheat the oven to 375°F.

Brush a baking dish with a little of the olive oil. Place the salmon fillets in the dish. Season with salt and pepper.

In a large bowl, combine the tomatoes, olives, garlic, lemon juice, capers, and sugar. Spoon the tomato mixture over the salmon fillets, then top with the bread crumbs. Drizzle with the remaining olive oil and bake for 15 minutes for medium-rare. Serve immediately.

Balsamic-Glazed Salmon

SERVES 4

Salmon is a rich and fatty fish that is popular with most dinner guests. When purchasing the fish, choose wild Pacific salmon whenever possible.

½ cup balsamic vinegar
1 tablespoon honey
Four 6-ounce salmon fillets
Iodized table salt and freshly ground black pepper
1 tablespoon olive oil

Mix together the vinegar and honey in a small bowl. Season the salmon fillets with salt and pepper; brush with the honey-balsamic glaze.

Heat the olive oil in a cast-iron skillet over medium-high heat. Sear the salmon fillets until lightly browned and medium rare in the center, 3 to 4 minutes per side.

Let sit for 5 minutes before serving.

Bouillabaisse

SERVES 8

Bouillabaisse is an aromatic seafood soup from Marseilles. Classic recipes call for a variety of seafood, so feel free to use what you can find—the results will still be delicious. Shellfish is especially good for the thyroid and can be enjoyed several times a week. Serve this hearty stew over brown rice.

½ cup olive oil
2 onions, diced
4 tomatoes, peeled and chopped
5 garlic cloves, minced
6 cups reduced-sodium fish stock
8 small red potatoes, cubed and cooked
1 cup dry white wine
1 bunch chopped fresh basil
1 tablespoon Tabasco or other hot sauce
1 teaspoon dried thyme
½ teaspoon powdered saffron
10 clams, scrubbed
10 mussels, scrubbed
1 pound medium shrimp, peeled and deveined
1 pound fresh monkfish fillets, cut into chunks
1 pound fresh cod, cut into chunks
½ cup chopped fresh flat-leaf parsley

Heat the olive oil in a large Dutch oven or stockpot over medium-high heat. Add the onions and cook until soft and translucent, about 5 minutes. Add the tomatoes and garlic, lower the heat, and simmer for 5 minutes more. Add the fish stock, potatoes, wine, basil, hot sauce, thyme, and saffron; simmer for 20 minutes.

Purée half of this mixture in the blender, then return it to the pot. (Alternatively, you can use a handheld immersion blender to purée some of the soup right in the pot.)

Add the shellfish, fish, and parsley and simmer for 20 minutes. Discard any clams or mussels that do not open.

Serve immediately.

Burgundy Salmon

SERVES 4

Although usually associated with beef, red wine complements the salmon in this dish perfectly. Use a high-quality wine that you would happily drink on its own. Wild salmon is a healthier choice for you and the environment than farmed Atlantic salmon. This simple preparation makes for an elegant dinner, even on weeknights.

Four 6-ounce salmon steaks

Iodized table salt and freshly ground black pepper

1 tablespoon olive oil

1 shallot, minced

2 cups Burgundy wine (Pinot Noir)

½ cup reduced-sodium beef broth

2 tablespoons tomato paste

1 teaspoon chopped fresh thyme, for garnish

Preheat the oven to 350°F.

Season the salmon steaks with salt and pepper. Wrap the steaks in aluminum foil and place on a baking sheet. Bake for 10 to 13 minutes.

Heat the olive oil in a deep skillet over medium heat. Add the shallot and cook until tender, about 3 minutes. Add the wine, beef broth, and tomato paste; simmer until the sauce thickens and reduces by one-third, about 10 minutes.

Plate the fish, pour the sauce over each steak, and garnish with the fresh thyme. Serve immediately.

Chermoula Salmon

SERVES 4

Chermoula is a traditional Moroccan marinade that is typically used with fish. With cilantro, a good source of phytonutrients, and parsley, which provides high levels of vitamin K, this exotic dish effectively boosts your health. The marinade keeps for up to a week in the refrigerator.

½ cup olive oil
½ cup chopped fresh cilantro
4 garlic cloves, minced
Juice of 1 lemon
1 tablespoon ground cumin
1 tablespoon red pepper flakes
1 tablespoon paprika
1 teaspoon iodized table salt
Four 6-ounce salmon fillets

Combine all the ingredients except the salmon in a small saucepan over medium heat. Heat until the mixture is hot, but do not let it boil. Remove the pan from the heat and let the marinade cool to room temperature.

Place the salmon fillets on a baking sheet and rub the marinade over them. Cover and refrigerate for at least 1 hour and up to 4 hours.

Preheat the oven to 450°F.

Bake until the salmon is medium-rare and slightly firm to the touch, 10 to 13 minutes. Serve immediately.

Hearty Clam Spaghetti

SERVES 4

This simple weeknight dish provides a surprising amount of iron, protein, omega-3 fatty acids, and vitamin B$_{12}$. Contrary to popular belief, clams have more iron than beef and as much protein as chicken. Leave out the bacon if you are trying to cut calories, but in that case you'll want to use a small amount of olive oil to cook the onion and green bell pepper.

4 ounces sliced bacon

1 medium onion, diced

1 medium green bell pepper, seeded and diced

4 garlic cloves, minced

½ cup fresh flat-leaf parsley, chopped

½ teaspoon cayenne pepper

Iodized table salt and freshly ground black pepper

1 pound whole-wheat spaghetti

3 dozen clams, scrubbed

½ cup dry white wine

1 lemon, cut into wedges, for serving

½ cup freshly grated low-fat Parmesan cheese, for serving

Heat a large skillet over medium heat. Add the bacon, onion, bell pepper, and garlic and cook until the bacon is slightly crisp and the onion is translucent, about 5 minutes. Add the parsley, cayenne pepper, season with salt and black pepper, and remove from the heat.

Cook the pasta according to the package directions, drain, and transfer to a large serving dish.

While the pasta is cooking, bring another large pot of water to a boil over high heat. Add the clams and boil until they open, about 10 minutes. Discard any that do not open. Remove the clams from the pot, reserving the water, and shell half of them.

Return the skillet with the bacon mixture to medium-high heat. Add the shelled clams to the skillet, along with the remaining clams in their shells, the white wine, and 2 cups of the liquid used to boil the clams. Stir to combine and heat through.

Ladle the clam mixture over the pasta and toss. Serve, offering lemon wedges and Parmesan cheese alongside.

Cod Gratin

A gratin is a tasty French preparation that usually involves a rich white sauce. In this recipe, cod, leeks, and onion play the feature role and peek out from a whole-wheat bread crumb crust. This recipe also works well with halibut.

½ cup olive oil
1 pound fresh cod
1 cup pitted, chopped black olives
4 leeks, white and light green parts, sliced
1 cup whole-wheat bread crumbs
¾ cup reduced-sodium chicken broth
Iodized table salt and freshly ground black pepper

Preheat the oven to 350°F.

Brush a baking dish with a little of the olive oil, lay the cod in it, and bake for 5 to 7 minutes. Cool and cut into 1-inch pieces.

Heat some of the remaining olive oil in a large skillet over medium-low heat. Add the olives and leeks and cook until the leeks are tender, about 10 minutes. Add the bread crumbs and chicken broth, stirring to mix. Gently fold in the pieces of cod.

Brush four individual gratin dishes with some more olive oil. Divide the cod mixture between the gratin dishes, and drizzle with the remaining olive oil. Season with salt and pepper.

Bake until warmed through, about 15 minutes. Serve immediately.

Grilled Herbed Tuna

SERVES 4

Tuna's meaty texture allows it to stand up to grilling, making it a nice alternative to hamburgers and hot dogs. Brush the grill grates with oil before adding the fish so it doesn't stick.

2 tablespoons olive oil
2 tablespoons chopped fresh basil
Juice and zest of 1 lemon
2 teaspoons chopped fresh cilantro
1 garlic clove, minced
Four 6-ounce tuna steaks
2 tablespoons chopped fresh flat-leaf parsley, for garnish
Iodized table salt and freshly ground black pepper

Preheat the grill to medium-high. Oil the grates.

Combine the oil, basil, lemon juice and zest, cilantro, and garlic in a small bowl. Place the tuna steaks on a plate and brush each side of the tuna with the mixture. Cover the plate and transfer to the refrigerator to marinate for at least 30 minutes and up to 4 hours.

Grill until medium-rare, turning halfway through the cooking time, 8 to 12 minutes, depending on the thickness.

Garnish with the chopped parsley, season with salt and pepper, and serve immediately.

Halibut with Roasted Vegetables

SERVES 6

Halibut can be served in a variety of ways and with different types of seasonings and vegetables. With traditional Mediterranean vegetables, it provides a great amount of nutrition—but feel free to improvise with what's available and fresh.

¼ cup button mushrooms, coarsely chopped
2 small tomatoes, coarsely chopped
1 small white onion, diced
2 zucchini, diced
2 garlic cloves, minced
1 teaspoon dried herbes de provence
½ cup olive oil
Iodized table salt and freshly ground black pepper
1½ pounds halibut steak, cut into 6 pieces
3 tablespoons finely chopped fresh tarragon
Juice of 1 lemon

Preheat the oven to 350°F.

Toss the mushrooms, tomatoes, onion, zucchini, garlic, and herbs on a large baking sheet with the olive oil; season with salt and pepper. Roast the vegetables until soft and slightly browned, 15 to 20 minutes. Be careful not to let them burn.

Meanwhile, place the halibut steaks on another baking sheet and season with the tarragon, more salt and pepper, and the lemon juice. Roast for 10 to 13 minutes.

Top the halibut steaks with the roasted vegetables and serve immediately.

Herb-Marinated Flounder

Although dried herbs work in many recipes, fresh herbs are much tastier. Fresh herbs are also a better source of antioxidants. Most herbs grow easily in a pot on your back step or even a sunny windowsill in your kitchen.

¼ cup olive oil

4 garlic cloves, smashed

½ cup fresh flat-leaf parsley, chopped

2 tablespoons chopped fresh rosemary

2 tablespoons chopped fresh thyme

2 tablespoons chopped fresh sage

2 tablespoons freshly grated lemon zest

Iodized table salt and freshly ground black pepper

Four 6-ounce flounder fillets

Preheat the oven to 350°F.

Place the olive oil, garlic, and herbs in a food processor and season with salt and pepper. Blend to form a thick paste.

Place the fillets on a baking sheet and brush the paste on them. Cover and refrigerate for at least 1 hour and up to 4 hours.

Bake until the flounder is slightly firm and opaque, 8 to 10 minutes. Season with salt and pepper and serve.

Poached Cod

SERVES 4

Poaching is a versatile technique for cooking soft fish, such as flounder and cod. This dish is both elegant and simple—ideal if you're entertaining on a weeknight. Serve with a simple salad.

1 tablespoon olive oil
½ cup thinly sliced onion
1 tablespoon minced garlic
One 14½-ounce can diced tomatoes, drained
2 cups reduced-sodium chicken broth
½ cup dry white wine
Juice and zest of 1 orange
Pinch of red pepper flakes
1 bay leaf
1 pound cod

Heat the olive oil in a large skillet. Add the onion and cook until translucent and soft, about 10 minutes. Add the garlic and cook for 1 minute. Add the tomatoes, chicken broth, wine, orange juice and zest, red pepper flakes, and bay leaf, and simmer for 5 minutes to meld the flavors.

Carefully add the fish in a single layer. Cover and simmer for 6 to 7 minutes.

Transfer the fish to a serving dish. Remove the bay leaf and ladle the remaining sauce over the fish. Serve immediately.

Roasted Sea Bass

SERVES 6

Roasting is an easy and forgiving way to prepare almost any fish. Use it to cook whole fish, fish fillets, or even fish chunks; simply adjust the cooking time based on the fish's size. Enjoy this dish with potatoes.

5 tablespoons olive oil

2 pounds whole sea bass or fillets

Iodized table salt and freshly ground black pepper

¼ cup dry white wine

1 tablespoon chopped fresh dill

2 teaspoons chopped fresh thyme

1 garlic clove, minced

Preheat the oven to 425°F.

Brush the bottom of a roasting pan with some of the olive oil. Place the fish in the pan and brush the fish with 3 tablespoons of the oil. Season with salt and pepper. Combine the remaining olive oil, wine, dill, thyme, and garlic in a small bowl and pour the mixture over the fish.

Bake until the flesh is firm and opaque, 10 to 15 minutes, depending on the size of the fish. Serve immediately.

Hearty Shrimp Salad

SERVES 4

Main-dish salads are a great way to get many servings of vegetables in one meal. Serve this tasty fare with whole-wheat pita bread for a light dinner.

2 tablespoons red wine vinegar
2 lemons
1 small shallot, finely minced
1 tablespoon chopped fresh mint
¼ teaspoon dried oregano
¼ cup olive oil
Iodized table salt and freshly ground black pepper
1 garlic clove, minced
1 pound shrimp, peeled and deveined
2 cups baby spinach leaves
1 cup chopped romaine lettuce
½ cup grape tomatoes
1 medium cucumber, peeled, seeded, and diced
½ cup pitted olives, chopped
¼ cup low-fat feta cheese

Combine the vinegar, juice of 1 lemon, shallot, mint, and oregano in a bowl. Add the olive oil, whisking constantly until you create a smooth emulsion, about 1 minute. Then season with salt and pepper. Cover the dressing and transfer to the refrigerator.

Combine the garlic with the juice of the other lemon and its zest in a shallow bowl or zipper-top plastic bag. Add the shrimp, cover the bowl or seal the bag, and transfer to the refrigerator for at least 2 hours or up to 4 hours.

Heat a grill or a frying pan over medium-high heat. Remove the shrimp from the marinade. Grill the shrimp in a grill basket or sauté in the frying pan until pink, 2 to 3 minutes.

In a large bowl toss the spinach, lettuce, tomatoes, cucumber, olives, and feta cheese together. Toss the shrimp with the salad mixture. Re-whisk the dressing and drizzle it over the salad. Serve immediately.

Eggplant and Tomato Ragu

Eggplant and tomatoes are common ingredients in Mediterranean cuisine. This hearty, versatile stew pairs well with crusty bread or pasta and is dense with nutrition.

Iodized table salt
1 large eggplant, peeled and cut in half
One 14½-ounce can diced tomatoes, undrained
1 cup reduced-sodium chicken broth
2 garlic cloves, smashed
1 tablespoon dried Italian seasoning blend
1 bay leaf
Freshly ground black pepper

Lightly salt the eggplant on both sides and let sit in a colander in the sink for 20 minutes to draw out the bitter juices. Rinse and pat dry with a paper towel. Dice the eggplant.

Put the eggplant, tomatoes with their juice, chicken broth, garlic, seasoning, and bay leaf in a large saucepan over high heat. Bring to a boil and reduce the heat to a simmer. Cover and simmer until the eggplant is tender, 30 to 40 minutes.

Remove the garlic cloves and bay leaf, season with salt and pepper, and serve.

Seasoned Root Vegetables

SERVES 4

Spices not only provide complex flavor but are also full of nutrients and antioxidant power. The slow cooking process develops a rich color and sweetness. A bowl of these hearty vegetables satisfies enough to serve as a meal.

2 medium carrots, peeled and cut into chunks

2 medium red or gold beets, cut into chunks

2 turnips, peeled and cut into chunks

2 tablespoons olive oil

1 teaspoon ground cumin

1 teaspoon sweet paprika

Iodized table salt and freshly ground black pepper

Juice of 1 lemon

1 small bunch chopped fresh flat-leaf parsley

Preheat the oven to 400°F.

Toss the vegetables with the olive oil and seasonings on a large baking sheet.

Spread the vegetables out in a single layer, sprinkle with the lemon juice, and roast until slightly browned and crisp, 30 to 40 minutes. Be careful not to let them burn.

Serve warm, topped with chopped parsley.

Dinner

Grilled Eggplant Pesto Stack

SERVES 4

This attractive eggplant stack is inspired by Italian cuisine. Although homemade pesto is not difficult to make, the store-bought variety will work if you're in a pinch. Eggplant really shines in this dish and is a useful substitute for meat.

1 large bunch fresh basil

½ cup pine nuts, toasted

2 or 3 garlic cloves

Juice of 1 lime

¾ cup plus 2 tablespoons olive oil

½ cup freshly grated low-fat Parmesan cheese

Iodized table salt and freshly ground black pepper

1 medium eggplant, sliced crosswise into ½-inch rounds

Put the basil, pine nuts, garlic, and lime juice in a food processor and pulse until a thick paste forms. With the machine running, slowly drizzle in ¾ cup of the olive oil through the feed tube, processing until creamy. Fold in the cheese. Season with salt and pepper.

Lightly salt the eggplant rounds and let rest for 20 minutes in a colander in the sink to draw out the bitter juices. Rinse the rounds and pat dry with a paper towel.

Preheat a grill to medium-high heat.

Brush the eggplant rounds with the remaining 2 tablespoons olive oil and grill, flipping once, until the rounds are lightly charred but still firm, 5 to 6 minutes per side.

On each plate, make a stack of eggplant rounds with pesto in between the layers. Serve warm.

Grilled Vegetables

Grilling vegetables instead of burgers or steaks is a great way to enjoy that smoky flavor without the extra fat and calories. Just a small amount of balsamic vinegar adds zing to a variety of grilled vegetables—choose your favorites and fire up that grill!

4 carrots, peeled and cut in half crosswise
2 onions, quartered
1 zucchini, cut crosswise into ½-inch rounds
1 red bell pepper, seeded and cut into squares
¼ cup olive oil, plus more for drizzling the vegetables
Iodized table salt and freshly ground black pepper
Balsamic vinegar

Heat the grill to medium-high.

Brush the vegetables lightly with the olive oil and season with salt and pepper. Place the carrots and onions on the grill first because they take the longest. After 3 to 4 minutes, add the zucchini and bell pepper to the grill. Cook the vegetables, turning once, for 3 to 4 minutes on each side.

Transfer to a serving dish, drizzle with a little more olive oil and a sprinkling of balsamic vinegar, and serve.

Dinner

Italian Mushroom-Stuffed Zucchini

SERVES 2

Seasoning vegetables with garlic, olive oil, parsley, and Italian herbs enriches the flavor, allowing you to enjoy food without excess calories. Serve this dish with a piece of fish for a delicious dinner.

2 tablespoons olive oil
2 cups finely chopped button mushrooms
2 garlic cloves, finely chopped
2 tablespoons reduced-sodium chicken broth
1 tablespoon finely chopped fresh flat-leaf parsley
1 tablespoon dried Italian seasoning blend
Iodized table salt and freshly ground black pepper
2 medium zucchini, cut in half lengthwise

Preheat the oven to 350°F.

Heat the olive oil in a large skillet over medium heat. Add the mushrooms and cook until tender, about 4 minutes. Add the garlic and cook for 2 minutes. Add the chicken broth and cook for another 3 minutes. Add the parsley and Italian seasoning and season with salt and pepper. Stir and remove from the heat.

Scoop out and discard the insides of the zucchini halves and stuff with the mushroom mixture. Place the zucchini halves in a casserole dish and pour in about 1 tablespoon of water just to coat the bottom of the dish. Cover with foil and bake until tender, 30 to 40 minutes.

Serve immediately.

Sweet Roasted Beet Salad with Oranges and Onions

SERVES 4

This sweet salad is a great source of phytonutrients, whether you serve it as a side or the main dish. For a heartier dinner, top with crumbled feta or goat cheese.

4 medium beets, trimmed and scrubbed
Juice and zest of 2 oranges
1 red onion, thinly sliced
2 tablespoons olive oil
1 tablespoon red wine vinegar
Juice of 1 lemon
Iodized table salt and freshly ground black pepper

Preheat the oven to 400°F.

Wrap the beets in foil and close tightly. Place them on a baking sheet and roast until tender enough to be pierced easily with a knife, about 40 minutes. Set aside until cool enough to handle. Cut into chunks.

Combine the beets with the orange juice and zest, red onion, olive oil, vinegar, and lemon juice. Season with salt and pepper and toss lightly.

Allow to sit at room temperature for 15 minutes for the flavors to meld before serving.

Dinner

Rosemary-Roasted Acorn Squash

SERVES 4

Acorn squash is a sweet, nutty winter squash. Acorn squash's fiber satisfies, and rosemary stimulates the immune system, increases circulation, and improves digestion.

1 acorn squash
2 tablespoons olive oil
2 tablespoons honey
2 tablespoons finely chopped fresh rosemary
Iodized table salt

Preheat the oven to 400°F.

Cut the squash in half and remove the seeds. Slice each half into 4 wedges.

Mix the olive oil, honey, and rosemary in a small bowl.

Lay the squash wedges on a baking sheet and brush one side with a bit of the olive oil mixture and season with salt. Turn the wedges over and do the same on the other side.

Bake, turning once, until the squash is tender and slightly caramelized, about 30 minutes. Serve immediately.

Stuffed Bell Peppers

Red bell peppers have more nutrients than green or yellow bell peppers, including plenty of vitamin C and carotenoids, and their nutritional value is best when they are not subjected to high heat. If you've already had your dairy allowance for the day, simply omit the cheese.

¾ cup feta cheese
½ cup pitted olives
½ cup plain Greek yogurt
¼ cup minced onion
¼ cup olive oil, plus more for drizzling
1 teaspoon finely chopped fresh thyme
½ teaspoon dried dill
Freshly ground pepper
6 bell peppers (any color), seeded and halved lengthwise

Combine all the ingredients except the bell peppers in a bowl.

Carefully spoon the mixture onto the bell pepper halves.

Refrigerate for at least 1 hour and up to 4 hours. Drizzle with olive oil before serving.

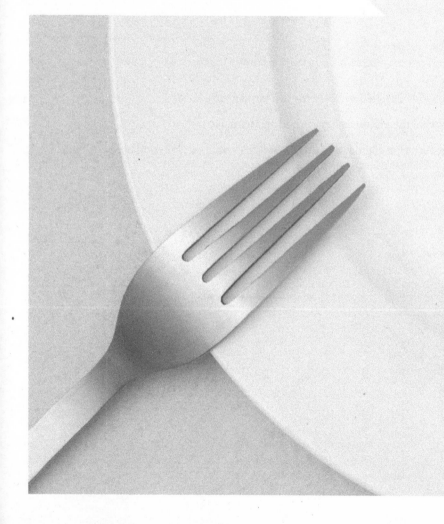

CHAPTER TEN

Savory Snacks

Stuffed Cucumbers

SERVES 2

Cucumbers contain a lot of water and also have antioxidant and anti-inflammatory properties. Combined with fresh tomato and avocado, this dish is nutrient dense. Enjoy this snack as a juicy summertime treat.

1 English cucumber
1 tomato, diced
1 avocado, peeled, pitted, and diced
Dash of lime juice
Iodized table salt and freshly ground black pepper
2 tablespoons chopped fresh cilantro, for garnish

Cut the cucumber in half lengthwise and scoop the flesh and seeds into a small bowl. Without mashing too much, gently combine the cucumber flesh and seeds with the tomato, avocado, and lime juice. Season with salt and pepper.

Put the mixture back into the cucumber halves and cut each piece in half crosswise. Garnish with the cilantro and serve.

111

Anchovy and Red Bell Pepper Antipasto

SERVES 4

Although "antipasto" means "before the meal," this delicious snack is good at any time of day. When bland crackers and cheese are not enough to satisfy your hunger, prepare this savory dish. The strong flavors are more satisfying, and you won't need to stuff yourself. Serve with whole-grain bread sticks or bread toasted with olive oil.

4 red bell peppers, halved lengthwise and seeded
One 6-ounce can anchovies in oil, drained and chopped
1 small shallot, minced
2 tablespoons capers, rinsed and drained
1 cup kalamata olives, pitted and chopped
½ cup olive oil
Iodized table salt and freshly ground black pepper

Preheat the broiler. Place the bell peppers on a baking sheet, cut-sides down. Broil until the skins blacken and blister, 5 to 10 minutes. Transfer the peppers to a paper bag. Seal and set aside to cool.

Take the peppers out of the bag and peel off the skins under running water, then pat dry with paper towels. Chop the peppers.

Combine the peppers, anchovies, shallot, capers, olives, and olive oil in a large bowl. Season with salt and pepper and serve.

Classic Hummus

This creamy and delicious dip can be served as an appetizer at a party or just as a snack. Hummus can also be used on sandwiches as a flavorful and healthy alternative to mayonnaise. Serve with fresh veggies or whole-wheat pita wedges.

3 cups cooked or canned chickpeas, rinsed and drained
¼ cup olive oil
Juice of 2 lemons
2 or 3 garlic cloves
¾ cup tahini (sesame paste)
Iodized table salt and freshly ground black pepper
½ cup pine nuts, toasted, for garnish (optional)
¼ cup chopped fresh flat-leaf parsley, for garnish

Heat the chickpeas slightly in the microwave. Combine the warm chickpeas, olive oil, lemon juice, and garlic in a food processor and purée until smooth. Add the tahini and continue to blend until creamy. If it is too thick, add a bit of water to thin it out. Season with salt and pepper and remove from the food processor to a serving bowl.

Garnish with the pine nuts, if desired, and the chopped parsley. Serve.

113

Savory Snacks

Marinated Olives and Mushrooms

A dish full of marinated olives and mushrooms is always a success at a party. The tangy and salty olives combine with mild button mushrooms to create a delicious snack to eat while mingling. These savory treats are simple and easy to prepare. Make ahead of time and store in the refrigerator for up to 3 days. Serve at room temperature.

1 pound small white button mushrooms
1 pound mixed olives
1 tablespoon white wine vinegar
2 tablespoons fresh thyme
½ tablespoon crushed fennel seeds
Pinch of red pepper flakes
Olive oil, to cover
Iodized table salt and freshly ground black pepper

Combine the mushrooms, olives, vinegar, thyme, fennel seeds, and red pepper flakes in a glass jar or other airtight container. Cover with olive oil and season with salt and pepper. Shake to distribute the ingredients.

Allow to marinate for at least 1 hour. Serve at room temperature.

Mini Greek Lettuce Wraps

SERVES 6

This bite-size snack is easy to assemble and very versatile. Swap the tomatoes, cucumbers, and red onion for any vegetables you like. Tuck away in a plastic container in the refrigerator or double the recipe and serve as an elegant, nutritious appetizer.

½ tomato, diced
½ cucumber, diced
½ red onion, sliced
½ ounce low-fat feta cheese, crumbled
Juice of ½ lemon
1½ teaspoons olive oil
Iodized table salt and freshly ground black pepper
6 small iceberg lettuce leaves

Combine the tomato, cucumber, onion, and feta in a bowl with the lemon juice and olive oil. Season with salt and pepper.

Gently fill each lettuce leaf with a tablespoon of the veggie mixture. Without tearing the lettuce, roll each leaf as tightly as you can. Lay the wraps, seam-sides down, on a plate.

Avocado and Asparagus Wraps

Avocados are not just for guacamole at parties—they provide a great addition to the diet because of their healthful fats. Use mashed avocados in place of mayonnaise in salads, sandwiches, and wraps. This wrap works nicely as a healthy snack.

12 asparagus spears, trimmed
1 ripe avocado, peeled and pitted
Juice of 1 lime
2 garlic cloves, minced
2 cups cooked brown rice, chilled
3 tablespoons plain Greek yogurt
Iodized table salt and freshly ground black pepper
Three 8-inch whole-grain tortillas
½ cup chopped fresh cilantro
2 tablespoons diced red onion

Steam the asparagus in the microwave or in a stovetop steamer until tender.

Mash the avocado, lime juice, and garlic in a medium bowl. In a separate medium bowl, mix the rice and yogurt. Season both mixtures with salt and pepper.

Heat the tortillas in the microwave or in a dry nonstick skillet.

Spread each tortilla with some of the avocado mixture and top with the rice mixture, cilantro, and onion, followed by 4 asparagus spears.

Fold in both sides of the tortilla, then roll tightly to close. Cut in half diagonally before serving.

Mini Moroccan Pumpkin Cakes

SERVES 6

Pumpkin is a popular ingredient in Moroccan dishes. This exotic dish is a tasty way to contribute to your daily requirement of protein. Serve these spicy panfried cakes with a side of tzatziki or Greek yogurt. (Make sure to allow time in between taking thyroid medication and consuming walnuts, as they interfere with certain medications.)

2 cups cooked brown rice
1 cup canned pumpkin purée
½ cup finely chopped walnuts
3 tablespoons olive oil
½ medium onion, diced
½ red bell pepper, seeded and diced
1 teaspoon ground cumin
Iodized table salt and freshly ground black pepper
1 teaspoon hot paprika or pinch of cayenne

Combine the rice, pumpkin, and walnuts in a large bowl; set aside.

In a small skillet, heat 1 tablespoon of the olive oil over medium heat. Add the onion and bell pepper and cook until soft, about 5 minutes. Stir in the cumin.

Add the onion mixture to the rice mixture. Mix thoroughly and season with salt, pepper, and paprika.

In a large skillet, heat the remaining 2 tablespoons of olive oil over medium heat.

Form the rice mixture into six 1-inch-thick patties and add them to the skillet. Cook until both sides are browned and crispy. Serve immediately.

Roasted Eggplant Dip with Spicy Yogurt Sauce

SERVES 8

This dish is heavily influenced by Mediterranean cuisine. The eggplant dip is a take on the traditional baba ghanoush and the yogurt dip resembles Greek tzatziki. Serve with raw vegetables or toasted pita.

Iodized table salt
2 large eggplants, peeled and cut in half
1 cup plain Greek yogurt
½ cucumber, grated
2 tablespoons chopped fresh dill
1 jalapeño pepper, seeded and chopped
6 garlic cloves, minced
Freshly ground black pepper
Juice of 2 lemons
2 red bell peppers, diced
2 cups diced tomatoes
20 yellow or red cherry tomatoes
½ cup chopped fresh flat-leaf parsley
¼ cup chopped fresh chives
3 leaves fresh basil, thinly sliced
1 tablespoon olive oil

Preheat the oven to 450°F.

Lightly salt the eggplants on both sides and let sit in a colander in the sink for 20 minutes to draw out the bitter juices. Rinse and pat dry with a paper towel.

Transfer the eggplants to a baking sheet and roast until they fall apart, about 35 minutes. Set aside until cool enough to handle.

While the eggplant is roasting. Mix the yogurt, cucumber, dill, jalapeño, and 1 of the minced garlic cloves in a small bowl. Season with salt and pepper. Cover and refrigerate until serving time.

Scoop the eggplant flesh into a strainer. Discard the skins.

Drizzle the eggplant flesh with the lemon juice, then squeeze out the moisture by pressing on the eggplant flesh with the back of a spoon.

Chop the eggplant and combine it in a large bowl with the bell peppers, tomatoes, remaining 5 minced garlic cloves, parsley, chives, basil, and olive oil. Season with salt and pepper.

Serve the eggplant dip and the yogurt sauce side by side.

Cucumber-Basil Sandwiches

SERVES 2

Not only does the basil add flavor to this hummus sandwich, but it is also rich in antioxidants. Do not remove the skin or seeds of the cucumber because both contain many nutrients. The sandwich is good served open-faced, if you wish to cut down on calories and carbohydrates.

4 slices whole-grain bread
¼ cup Classic Hummus (see p. 113) or purchased hummus
1 English cucumber, thinly sliced
4 leaves fresh basil

Spread the hummus on 2 slices of bread and layer the cucumber slices onto it. Top with the basil leaves and close the sandwiches. Press down lightly and serve immediately.

Spicy Black Bean Dip

YIELDS 2 CUPS

Black beans are a great way to get your protein without eating meat. Enjoy this dip as a snack with vegetable sticks.

2 garlic cloves, peeled
Juice of 1 lime
2 tablespoons water
1 tablespoon tomato paste
1 teaspoon ground cumin
1 teaspoon chili powder
½ teaspoon hot sauce
¼ teaspoon ground ginger
¼ teaspoon iodized table salt
¼ cup chopped fresh cilantro or basil
2 scallions, sliced
One 19-ounce can black beans, rinsed and drained
1 cup coarsely chopped tomato

In a small saucepan of simmering water, blanch the garlic cloves for 3 minutes. Drain well.

In a food processor, combine the blanched garlic, lime juice, water, tomato paste, cumin, chili powder, hot sauce, ginger, and salt; process until blended.

Add the cilantro (or basil), scallions, and beans and pulse until combined but still chunky.

Transfer the dip to a serving bowl, stir in the tomato, and serve.

Sesame Cucumber "Noodles"

The soy sauce and sesame seeds keep this refreshing, low-calorie dish from being bland in taste or texture. Serve as a side dish or pack in a plastic container for a snack at work.

1 teaspoon light sesame seeds
1 teaspoon dark sesame seeds
2 medium cucumbers
1 tablespoon toasted sesame oil
2 tablespoon dark soy sauce
Red pepper flakes (optional)

Toast the light and dark sesame seeds in a dry skillet over medium heat until lightly golden.

Peel the cucumbers and cut off the ends. Using the julienne blade on a mandoline, run the cucumbers lengthwise to form flat "noodles." Rotate the cucumber as you go until you reach the seeds. (If you find it difficult to work with the whole cucumber, cut it in half to make it easier to handle.)

Place the cucumbers in a serving bowl and toss with the sesame oil, soy sauce, and 1 teaspoon of the mixed toasted sesame seeds.

Top with the rest of the sesame seeds and the red pepper flakes, if desired. Serve cold.

Pumpkin Power Snacks

Not only is this snack nutrition rich, but it also does not require baking! Pumpkins are loaded with fiber, which makes you feel fuller longer and keeps you from overeating. Pumpkins pack more potassium than bananas and help you restore electrolytes after a hard workout.

1 packed cup chopped dates
¼ cup honey
¼ cup canned pumpkin purée
1 tablespoon ground cinnamon
½ teaspoon ground ginger
¼ teaspoon ground nutmeg
Pinch of iodized table salt
1 cup old-fashioned oats
1 cup unsweetened shredded coconut, toasted
1 cup pumpkin seeds, toasted

Combine the dates, honey, pumpkin, cinnamon, ginger, nutmeg, and salt in a food processor and pulse until smooth and combined.

Transfer the mixture to a large bowl and stir in the oats, coconut, and pumpkin seeds. Cover and refrigerate for at least 30 minutes.

Once the mixture is cool, use a spoon to shape it into 1-inch balls. Alternatively, you can line a small baking sheet with parchment paper, press the mixture evenly into the pan, chill, and then cut into bars.

Store, covered, in the refrigerator for up to 2 weeks.

Toasted Nori Chips

SERVES 4

Nori, a type of seaweed, is a wonderful source of iodine as well as omega-3 acids. The iodine helps the thyroid function, and omega-3 acids are good for both skin and heart health. You can find nori sheets at Asian grocery stores, health food stores, and some large supermarkets.

8 nori sheets
Iodized table salt
Toasted sesame oil

Preheat the oven to 250°F.

Brush or spray each sheet of nori very lightly with a little water and season it with salt. Fold each sheet in half and press the sides together.

Use a pizza cutter or sharp knife to cut the doubled nori sheets into 1-by-3-inch strips.

Transfer the strips to a baking sheet in a single layer. Bake until dark and crisp, 15 to 20 minutes.

When the chips are done, carefully slide them onto racks to cool. Brush the chips gently with sesame oil and serve. Or, if you're not going to serve them right away, leave off the oil and store the chips in a covered container for up to 2 days, then add the oil when ready to serve.

Artichoke-Chickpea Salad

SERVES 4

This salad features Mediterranean ingredients, including artichoke hearts and chickpeas. The sun-dried tomatoes provide a strong flavor. Chickpeas are rich in fiber and protein, and artichokes provide a great amount of antioxidants, making this a well-rounded snack.

One 15-ounce can artichoke hearts, rinsed, drained, and chopped
One 15-ounce can chickpeas, rinsed and drained
1 tablespoon chopped sun-dried tomatoes
3 tablespoons prepared red pesto

In a large bowl, mix all the ingredients until well combined. Serve immediately or store in a covered container in the refrigerator for up to 2 days.

Deviled Eggs

SERVES 6

Deviled eggs are a Southern delicacy and common at picnics and parties. This simple recipe is for a less decadent version of deviled eggs that makes a great snack.

6 eggs
2 teaspoon yellow mustard
2 tablespoons light mayonnaise
Iodized table salt and freshly ground black pepper
Paprika (optional)

Place the eggs in a pot, cover with water, and bring to a boil over high heat. Boil for 5 minutes, then remove from the heat and let the eggs sit in the hot water for 15 minutes.

Remove the eggs and run cold water over them until cool enough to handle. Peel the eggs and slice in half lengthwise.

Dig out the egg yolks and empty into a bowl. Using a fork, mash the yolks with the mustard and mayonnaise; season with salt and pepper.

Spoon the egg yolk mixture back into the halved eggs. Sprinkle with paprika, if desired. Place on a plate, cover, and transfer to the refrigerator until chilled. Serve.

Carrot and Raisin Salad

SERVES 4

This light salad is rich in texture and abundant with nutrients. Carrots are a great source of antioxidants that protect against heart disease, improve vision, and have anti-aging effects on skin. High in fiber and low in calories, raisins give you a feeling of fullness without overeating.

6 medium carrots
⅓ cup golden raisins
Juice of 1 lemon
½ teaspoon iodized table salt
½ teaspoon freshly ground black pepper
1 teaspoon chopped fresh flat-leaf parsley, for garnish (optional)

Peel the carrots and shred on a box grater or in a food processor. Mix the carrots with the raisins in a medium bowl.

In a separate bowl, whisk the lemon juice with the salt and pepper. Toss the carrots and raisins with the lemon juice mixture.

Garnish with the parsley, if desired, and serve.

White Bean Bruschetta

SERVES 4

Bruschetta is an Italian antipasto that in its simplest form consists of grilled bread, garlic, and olive oil. This version adds a little heartiness to the antipasto with the addition of cannellini beans. These beans are an inexpensive staple filled with protein and fiber.

2 tablespoons olive oil, divided
1 garlic clove, minced
One 15-ounce can cannellini beans, rinsed and drained
1 small baguette, cut into 1-inch-thick slices
Iodized table salt and freshly ground black pepper

Preheat the broiler.

In a small skillet, heat 1 tablespoon of the olive oil and the garlic. Add the beans and heat through, about 1 minute. Remove from the heat.

Brush the baguette slices with the remaining 1 tablespoon olive oil. Broil until golden and crisp, 30 to 60 seconds.

Top the baguette slices with the cannellini beans. Season with salt and pepper. Serve warm.

Summer Salsa

This salsa makes use of copious amounts of vegetables, giving you the vitamins and minerals you need to live a healthy lifestyle. With a beautiful array of colors, this dish is pleasing to the eye as well as the palate. Feel free to substitute whatever summer vegetables you have from the farmers' market or garden.

4 tomatoes, diced
2 red bell peppers, seeded and diced
2 green bell peppers, seeded and diced
1 cup diced zucchini
1 cup chopped red onion
1 cup cooked or canned black beans, rinsed and drained
½ cup chopped fresh cilantro
2 garlic cloves, minced
Juice of 2 limes
2 teaspoons sugar
1½ teaspoons seeded, finely chopped jalapeño pepper
1 teaspoon freshly ground black pepper
½ teaspoon iodized table salt
Whole-wheat chips, for serving

In a large bowl, combine all the ingredients except the chips. Toss gently to mix. Cover and refrigerate at least 30 minutes to blend flavors. Serve with the chips.

White Bean and Artichoke Dip

YIELDS 2 CUPS

This dip is low-fat and nutrient dense and very easy to make using staples that should stock the shelves of every kitchen cabinet. Not only is this dip simple, but it's a crowd-pleaser as well.

One 15-ounce can cannellini beans, rinsed and drained

One 14-ounce can artichoke hearts, rinsed and drained

1 garlic clove

2 tablespoons freshly squeezed lemon juice

1 teaspoon dried rosemary

Pinch of cayenne pepper (optional)

Pita chips, for serving

Place the cannellini beans, artichoke hearts, garlic, and lemon juice in a food processor. Blend until thick. Add the rosemary and blend in briefly.

Spoon the dip into a medium bowl. Sprinkle with cayenne pepper, if desired. Serve with the pita chips.

Salmon Salad and Nori Sheet Roll

SERVES 1

The salmon and nori provide a great amount of iodine and omega-3 acids, making this a fantastic snack for people with underactive thyroids. Nori sheets are usually sold in packs of 12 at the grocery store.

1 cup canned salmon
1 tablespoon freshly squeezed lemon juice
1 teaspoon minced red onion
1 nori sheet

Combine the salmon, lemon juice, and onion in a small bowl. Spoon the mixture evenly over the nori sheet. Roll up and serve.

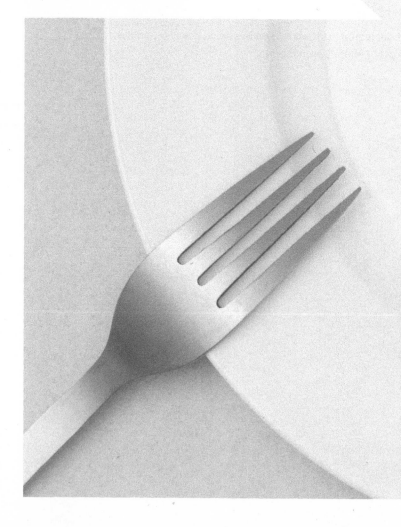

CHAPTER ELEVEN

Desserts

Balsamic Strawberries

This classic Italian treat is a great showcase for fresh strawberries and is a lovely way to clean the palate after dinner. The balsamic vinegar provides a strong and interesting contrast with the sweetness of the berries. Be sure to allow the strawberries to sit for a few minutes.

2 cups strawberries, hulled and sliced
2 tablespoons sugar
2 tablespoons balsamic vinegar

Put the strawberries in a bowl, sprinkle with the sugar, and lightly drizzle with the balsamic vinegar.

Toss to combine and let sit for about 10 minutes before serving.

Banana Cream Pie Parfaits

SERVES 2

The walnuts and banana in this dish provide potassium and omega-3 fatty acids. With low-fat vanilla pudding and graham cracker crumbs, this parfait is sweet but not decadent. These healthy parfaits can be prepared ahead of time. (Make sure to allow time in between taking thyroid medication and consuming walnuts, as they interfere with certain medications.)

1 cup low-fat vanilla pudding

2 reduced-sugar graham crackers, crushed

1 banana, peeled and sliced

¼ cup chopped walnuts

Honey, for drizzling

In two small parfait dishes or wine glasses, layer the ingredients, starting with the pudding and ending with the chopped walnuts. You can repeat the layers, depending on the size of the glass and your preferences. Transfer to the refrigerator to chill.

Drizzle with the honey and serve.

Berry Crumble

SERVES 6

Traditionally a decadent dessert, this version is loaded with antioxidant-filled berries and cholesterol-lowering oats. The frozen berries make this dish convenient all year round. If you do not have a cast-iron skillet, a casserole dish will work as well.

3 cups frozen mixed berries
1 cup rolled oats
2 tablespoons brown sugar
1 tablespoon whole-wheat flour
2 tablespoons butter, cut into little chunks

Preheat the oven to 400°F.

In a 10-inch cast-iron skillet, lay the berries in an even layer.

Mix the oats with the sugar and flour in a small bowl. Spread the oat mixture evenly on top of the berries.

Scatter the butter chunks on top and bake until the top is brown and the berries are bubbly, 40 to 50 minutes.

Serve warm.

Cocoa and Coconut Banana Slices

SERVES 1

Frozen bananas have a creamy consistency that mimics ice cream. Bananas are good for you, too, providing dietary fiber, vitamin C, potassium, and manganese. This dessert makes a great snack for adults and kids alike.

1 banana, sliced
1 tablespoon shredded unsweetened coconut
½ teaspoon unsweetened cocoa powder
Honey

Lay the banana slices on a parchment-lined baking sheet in a single layer.

Put the sheet in the freezer until the banana is firm but not frozen solid, about 10 minutes.

Mix the coconut with the cocoa powder in a small bowl.

Dip the banana slices in the honey, then in the coconut and cocoa powder mixture.

Eat immediately.

Cucumber-Lime Pops

Pops are classic summer treats that everyone finds hard to resist. Cucumbers have both antioxidant and anti-inflammatory properties, making this a healthy alternative to store-bought pops. Keep some of these refreshing and healthy pops in the freezer and enjoy them all summer long.

2 cups cold water
1 cucumber, peeled
¼ cup honey
Juice of 1 lime

In a blender, purée the water, cucumber, honey, and lime juice. Pour into pop molds, freeze, and enjoy on a hot day.

Figs with Chocolate Sauce

SERVES 4

Desserts in the Mediterranean need not be complicated. The combination of fruit and chocolate is a simple concept with serious taste. This easy treat would be a good snack, too. You could also serve it with Greek yogurt.

¼ cup honey
1 teaspoon unsweetened cocoa powder
4 fresh figs

Combine the honey and cocoa powder in a small bowl and mix well to form syrup.

Cut the figs in half and place on plates, cut-sides up. Drizzle with the syrup and serve.

Blueberry Mousse

SERVES 6

Blueberry mousse is a perfectly refreshing dessert for summer. Blueberries are abundant in antioxidants and helpful at reducing symptoms of hypothyroidism. The antioxidants also help renew the skin and keep you looking younger!

1 cup blueberries
½ cup sugar
5 tablespoons water
¾ teaspoon unflavored gelatin
Pinch of iodized table salt
2 egg whites
¼ teaspoon pure vanilla extract
Whipping cream

Toss the blueberries with 1 tablespoon of the sugar in the bowl of a food processor. Let stand for 10 minutes. Process until smooth.

Pour 2 tablespoons of the water into the bowl of a stand mixer fitted with a paddle and sprinkle with the gelatin. Let stand for 5 minutes.

Place 6 tablespoons of the sugar, the remaining 3 tablespoons water, and a pinch of salt in a small heavy saucepan. Bring to a boil over medium-high heat, stirring until the sugar dissolves. Cook, without stirring, until a candy thermometer registers 240°F, about 4 minutes.

Meanwhile, add the egg whites to the gelatin mixture. Beat on high speed until foamy. Gradually add the remaining 1 tablespoon sugar, continuing to beat at high speed until soft peaks form.

Gradually pour the hot sugar syrup into the egg white mixture, beating first at medium speed and then at high speed until stiff peaks form again. Beat in the vanilla.

Place the cream in a clean mixing bowl. Beat at high speed until stiff peaks form. Gently fold one-fourth of the egg white mixture into the whipping cream. Fold in the remaining egg white mixture. Fold in the blueberry mixture.

Spoon about ½ cup mousse into each of six dessert glasses. Chill for 2 hours or until set. Serve chilled.

Glossary

Allergen: A substance that causes an immune system reaction in the body because it is perceived as foreign. The body then releases chemicals to attempt to neutralize the substance. This causes inflammation.

BMI: Body mass index. BMI is the proportion of fat to muscle in your body.

Calorie: A unit of energy from food that must be expended or it will be stored as fat.

Carbohydrates: Foods containing starch (breads, cereals) or simple sugars (candy) that are easily broken down into blood glucose by your body.

Cortisol: A hormone released by the adrenal glands in time of stress to help the body preserve its energy and use its fuel to fight stress. Cortisol suppresses "nonessential" processes like digestion and the immune system so your body can fight the immediate "threat" by providing energy (glucose) to your heart and brain.

Enzymes: Proteins used by the body for important processes like digestion.

Fats: Compounds called lipids are usually divided into fats, which are solid at room temperature, and oils, which are liquid at room temperature. When taken as a nutrient, fats can be metabolized to blood glucose. Fat in the body also stores energy in a form that can be later broken down by the body into blood glucose. Fats are needed by the body for structure and metabolism.

Genetics: The influence of inherited traits on your body. Genetic traits can often be modified by the environment.

Glycemic index: A measure of how quickly blood sugar rises after eating a particular food.

Hormones: Chemical "messengers" sent by glands throughout your body. Hormones reach your body's cells and influence how they work.

Inflammation: The body's response to perceived injury or foreign substance. The body tries to neutralize or destroy the foreign substance by producing chemicals, which may cause irritation of the body's tissues.

Insulin: A hormone released by the pancreas that helps your body's cells take up glucose.

Lipids: Naturally occurring molecules that include fats.

Metabolism: The process through which the body breaks down your nutritional intake into parts and rebuilds the components into the substances you need to maintain your health.

Minerals: Naturally occurring substances that are not made of carbon, hydrogen, nitrogen, and oxygen. Certain minerals are necessary for health and must be taken in through the diet. Selenium and iodine are examples of two minerals important for thyroid function.

Nutrients: Chemicals that must be taken from the environment and processed by an organism in order to survive.

Proteins: Large biological molecules used in your body to renew its structure and to create chemical messengers like hormones and neurotransmitters. Proteins are made up of amino acids, smaller molecules that come from the proteins you eat. Meats, fish, eggs, dairy products, soy, and legumes are rich sources of proteins.

Thyroid: An important gland in your body that regulates metabolism by sending hormones to act upon cells in the body.

T3: Triiodothyronine. The most potent thyroid hormone, T3 has an effect that is four times as strong as that of T4 on the body's cells. T3 is the active thyroid hormone and is released by the thyroid gland. It has effects on every cell in the body, with the function of regulating metabolism, body temperature, heart rate, and development. T3 is released in response to high levels of TSH released by the pituitary gland.

T4: Thyroxine. T4 is a precursor to T3, which is formed by removing an iodine atom from T4.

TSH: Thyroid-stimulating hormone. TSH is released by the pituitary gland in the presence of low levels of circulating thyroid hormone. TSH signals the thyroid gland to produce more thyroid hormone. When there is enough thyroid hormone, the pituitary gland stops producing TSH, creating a feedback loop.

Vitamins: Compounds necessary for an organism that cannot be synthesized within the organism and must be taken in through diet.

References

Braverman, L. E., & Cooper, D. S. (2012). *Werner & Ingbar's the Thyroid: A Fundamental and Clinical Text*. Philadelphia: Lippincott Williams & Wilkins.

Bunevičius, R.; Kažanavičius, G.; Žalinkevičius, R.; & Prange, A. J. (1999). Effects of Thyroxine as Compared with Thyroxine plus Triiodothyronine in Patients with Hypothyroidism. *New England Journal of Medicine*. doi: 10.1056/NEJM199902113400603.

Gharib, H.; Tuttle, R. M.; Baskin, H. J.; Fish, L. H.; Singer, P. A.; & McDermott, M. T. (2005). Consensus Statement: Subclinical Thyroid Dysfunction: A Joint Statement on Management from the American Association of Clinical Endocrinologists, the American Thyroid Association, and the Endocrine Society. *Journal of Clinical Endocrinology & Metabolism*. doi: 10.1210/jc.2004-1869.

Nygaard, B.; Jensen, E. W.; Kvetny, J.; Jarlov, A.; & Faber, J. (2009). Effect of combination therapy with thyroxine (T4) and 3,5,3'-triiodothyronine versus T4 monotherapy in patients with hypothyroidism, a double-blind, randomised cross-over study. *European Journal of Endocrinology*. doi:10.1530/EJE-09-0542.

Recipe Index

Printed in April 2023
by Rotomail Italia S.p.A., Vignate (MI) - Italy